I WANT A CHRISTIAN PSYCHIATRIST

Also by David Enoch

Healing the Hurt Mind (11th Edition)
Uncommon Psychiatric Syndromes (4th Edition)
Schizophrenia: Voices in the Dark (with Mary Moate) *(2nd Edition)*
Psychiatric Disorders in Dental Practice (with Robert Jagger)

I WANT A CHRISTIAN PSYCHIATRIST

FINDING A PATH BACK TO SPIRITUAL AND MENTAL WHOLENESS

DR DAVID ENOCH

MONARCH
BOOKS

Oxford, UK & Grand Rapids, Michigan

First published in the UK in 2006 by Monarch Books
(a publishing imprint of Lion Hudson plc),
Mayfield House, 256 Banbury Road, Oxford OX2 7DH.
Tel: +44 (0)1865 302750 Fax: +44 (0)1865 302757
Email: monarch@lionhudson.com
www.lionhudson.com

ISBN-13: 978-1-85424-684-4 (UK)
ISBN-10: 1-85424-684-4 (UK)
ISBN-13: 978-0-8254-6143-9 USA)
ISBN-10: 0-8254-6143-X (USA)

Distributed by:
UK: Marston Book Services Ltd, PO Box 269,
Abingdon, Oxon OX14 4YN;
USA: Kregel Publications, PO Box 2607,
Grand Rapids, Michigan 49501.

Unless otherwise stated, Scripture quotations are taken from The New Revised Standard Version, Anglicised Edition, copyright 1989, 1995 by the Division of Christian Education of the National Council of the Churches of Christ in the United States of America, and are used by permission. All rights reserved.

Thankyou Music/Adm. by worshiptogether.com songs excl. UK & Europe, adm. by kingswaysongs.com tym@kingsway.co.uk. Used by permission.

The text paper used in this book has been made from wood independently certified as having come from sustainable forests.

British Library Cataloguing Data
A catalogue record for this book is available from the British Library.

Printed and bound in Reading by Cox & Wyman Ltd.

To Anne

CONTENTS

Acknowledgments

In writing this book I am much indebted to a number of people. Tony Collins' (Editorial Director, Monarch Books) trust in me is deeply appreciated – as is his enthusiastic support and keen intellect, which demands clarity and focus from his authors. My thanks to Simon Cox, Project Editor for his empathic encouragement and assiduousness.

I have been fortunate to work with a superb editorial consultant, Jan Greenough, whose sensitivity, spirituality and precision has made a big difference to this book.

I thank my wife Anne, to whom I dedicate this book, for her loving assiduous support and wise suggestions which she will no doubt recognize in certain chapters.

Finally, I must thank my colleagues, friends and especially those whom I have been privileged to treat and minister to for all they have taught me and which I have been able to share in this book, with the hope that many readers will thus be led back to a pathway of mental and spiritual wholeness.

Preface

One Sunday afternoon last month, for what seemed like the thousandth time in my long career, I had a phone call from someone saying, "I want to see a Christian psychiatrist."

This time it was a father anxious about his son; on other occasions it has been someone looking for help for a mother, father, brother, sister, grandparent, friend, fellow church member or spouse. As usual, the family were facing an acute crisis which had driven them to seek help, yet the father was very reluctant to admit that his son needed psychiatric care or treatment.

"He's not really ill," he said, "just a bit low."

All kinds of euphemisms are used to describe people's mental state: from depression to schizophrenia, even the names of mental illnesses seem to strike fear into people's hearts, so they avoid them the way people used to avoid mentioning cancer.

My caller then became prescriptive.

"I don't want you to diagnose a mental illness," he said. "And I don't want you to prescribe any drugs. Just tell us what would be the best way to help him. Will it be all right if I bring him in to see you tomorrow?"

I always think this is extraordinary. People wouldn't dream of going to their GP and telling him that he shouldn't diagnose cancer. Nor would they tell the surgeon not to operate on a tumour. Yet patients (or their relatives) who consult me for my professional expertise nevertheless regularly tell me what messages they do not want to hear, and what prescriptions they do not wish to receive.

These telephone calls tell me a great deal. Firstly, that there is still in the general population a great fear of psychiatry as a profession, and that this fear is even worse among Christians. They ask for a Christian psychiatrist because they think they can trust a Christian more, or because they think that a Christian will understand their specific confusion between mental and spiritual well-being. Secondly, the caller has a fear of mental illness and the stigma it carries in our society – even more so among Christians. And thirdly, he is suspicious of medication as a treatment for mental illness.

Of course, I agreed to see the patient and to offer a diagnosis and suggestions for his treatment – but I knew that I would have an uphill struggle to convince the concerned parent to accept my advice. I find it amazing that at the beginning of the twenty-first century, when information is freely available on every subject, there is still so much fear and ignorance surrounding mental illness.

This is particularly so when one considers what a universal experience mental illness is: one in four people in the UK will experience some kind of mental health problem. The Royal College of Psychiatry recently ran a campaign called "Changing Minds" – its subtitle was "Every Family in the Land", driving home the point that almost everyone knows or is related to someone who has experienced some form of mental illness.

So why are Christians, in particular, so reluctant to admit to mental illness, and what are the particular issues surrounding the subject for them? Why does such a stigma attach to it, and why do people find it so hard to understand? And why do churches find it so hard to support their members when they suffer from it?

This book aims to provide information and reassurance to Christians who are anxious about accepting psychiatric help, either for themselves or a loved one. It also offers suggestions on how churches and individual Christians can offer support to those suffering any kind of mental illness, and thus reduce the suffering of victims and families, and accelerate the process of healing.

1

CHRISTIANS AND MENTAL ILLNESS

Everyone gets ill from time to time. Most people have no problem about discussing their ailments: "I've had flu," "I broke my arm," "I've got gallstones and I'll have to have an operation." People are seldom concerned about admitting to suffering from any of these conditions. Yet many patients who receive a diagnosis of mental illness are likely to feel embarrassment, shame and a desire to keep the whole thing a secret as far as possible. Why?

The stigma of mental illness

The fact is that a stigma is attached to mental illness, and sufferers fear that their lives may become even more difficult if their condition is known. Friends may become distant or abandon them altogether; employers may be unwilling to offer jobs to those who admit to having mental health problems; it may even be difficult to get a mortgage or insurance once a history of mental illness is established. Sufferers come up against prejudice and discrimination in every area of their lives.

I once gave a lecture, in the course of which I mentioned the fact that every family included someone who suffered from some form of mental illness. Afterwards

I was approached by a distinguished figure who thanked me for my talk, but said she disagreed with me on one point. She then began a tirade on the subject, saying that no one in her family had ever suffered from mental illness, and no one was ever likely to do so. Her emphatic and excited manner, together with her insistence on taking the matter so personally, convinced me that there was indeed someone in her family who suffered in this way, and that she was quite unable to accept it.

Mental illness is still regarded with fear: nothing is so frightening as looking at a friend or family member and seeing a change in their personality, the essence of self. Someone who is depressed may appear sad and unresponsive; in the elated phase of manic depression they may be excitable or irritable; someone suffering from anxiety may be unable to calm their fears by any rational argument. People find it deeply disturbing to interact with someone who no longer seems rational; they fear unpredictable and bizarre behaviour, which is embarrassing; and they are likely to avoid them, which results in social exclusion for the sufferer.

Such responses are not helped by the media, which deal mainly in stereotypes. Films and plays tend to portray the mentally ill as dangerous and potentially violent, though in fact you are more likely to encounter physical violence outside a pub at closing time, from the binge drinkers who are so much more socially acceptable – or indeed in the home, where domestic violence continues to increase.

There are other prejudices which spring from ignorance: some disorders, like depression or anxiety, are regarded as indicating weakness of character or lack of willpower. Many people think of mental illness as incurable, in spite of the fact that many treatments are nowadays very effective, and many sufferers in any case may have long periods of normal behaviour. Yet the stigma of mental illness makes it harder for sufferers to seek help, and harder for their friends and family to support them.

The prevalence of mental illness

It is much easier to stigmatize a group of people when they are seen as "other" – a minority who are different from the rest of society. Yet mental illness is not rare: one in four of us will suffer from it at some point during our lifetime. The statistics[1] reveal the enormity of the situation:

- One in six people will experience depression at some point in their life (most commonly between the ages of twenty-five and forty-five).

- One in ten people will have a disabling anxiety disorder at some point.

- One in 100 will suffer from manic depression or schizophrenia.

- Eighteen per cent of women and 11 per cent of men have a neurotic disorder such as anxiety, depression, phobias and panic attacks.

- Men are three times as likely as women to have alcohol dependency, and twice as likely to be dependent on drugs.

This prevalence is what lay behind the subtitle of the Royal College of Psychiatrists' campaign "Changing Minds – Every Family in the Land". The idea that everyone has contact with someone who suffers from some form of mental illness is probably the most potent force for change. When a condition is seen as common, it becomes more possible for it to be accepted as part of normality.

The Christian sufferer

It must be emphasized that the Christian faith does not impart immunity from mental illness; Christians are ordinary men and women, made of the same stuff as the rest of humanity, and therefore they suffer in the same way from these conditions just as they do from viruses or cancer. Mental illness is democratic: it attacks everyone and is no respecter of class, creed, nationality or family. Christians cannot escape the blight or the stigma of it. I hasten to add that faith can help them to overcome mental illness and it can help to alleviate symptoms, but the mere fact of being a Christian does not protect against breakdowns.

We trust in the promise of God: "I will never leave you or forsake you" (Hebrews 13:5), yet we know that this does not mean that we will be protected from all the troubles and ills of life on earth. Rather, God promises that we will not be overwhelmed by them. When Jesus prayed in Gethsemane on the night that he was betrayed, he said, " 'Father, if you are willing, remove this cup from me; yet, not my will but yours be done.' Then an angel from heaven appeared to him and gave him strength" (Luke 22:42–43). God did not take away the challenge of Christ's suffering, but he gave him strength to bear it and to transform it into a blessing for others.

As followers of Christ our position is similar. We may pray fervently to be delivered from the illnesses that assail us, but we accept that it may be God's will that we endure them. We know that "God is faithful, and he will not let you be tested beyond your strength, but with the testing he will also provide the way out so that you may be able to endure it" (1 Corinthians 10:13). We do not welcome illness and suffering, but they are an inevitable part of our lives. Through our sufferings we may learn more about the power of the Holy Spirit to strengthen and sustain us.

In fact it does appear that Christians are more prone to certain mental illnesses than non-Christians, perhaps because we spend a great deal of time thinking about our own standards of behaviour. This is a good thing: without such self-awareness, we could hardly begin to find our way in the Christian life, or set ourselves goals for improvement. Nevertheless, there is an essential tension in Christian thinking: we know that we are saved by grace, but we measure ourselves by the standards of the commandments. These may be the ten rules given by God to Moses on Mount Sinai, or the summary of the law given us by Jesus: "You shall love the Lord your God with all your heart, and with all your soul, and with all your mind, and with all your strength... you shall love your neighbour as yourself" (Mark 12:30–31).

In all cases, the outcome is the same: "All have sinned and fall short of the glory of God" (Romans 3:23). We fail to live up to our aspirations and the teachings of our Lord. The next verse continues, "They are now justified by his grace as a gift," but many Christians are still acutely aware of their failure, and they feel correspondingly guilty, and reluctant to accept that God's promises are for them too.

Certainly it is a striking fact that the gospel of peace and love does not seem to be a help to hundreds of Christians. It may be that an awareness of their own lack of commitment, and the lack of a true relationship with the loving Lord that makes them feel guilty, encouraging emotional and psychological disturbance.

We know that "A good tree cannot bear bad fruit, nor can a bad tree bear good fruit... Thus you will know them by their fruits" (Matthew 7: 18, 20), and we are miserably conscious that too often the fruits of our own lives are not good. We are constantly aware of the need to curb our negative emotions and feelings, our tendency to be critical, to hate, resent or envy other people, and our reluctance to give up the lordship of our lives to God. This tension between our faith and our "works" points up our failure, and dwelling on this can encourage depression.

Some Christians may also be more likely to suffer from obsessive-compulsive disorder (OCD). Paul tells us that the old rules have been superseded: "For the law of the Spirit of life in Christ Jesus has set you free from the law of sin and death" (Romans 8:2), yet we often feel safer if we set standards and rules for ourselves. People who are susceptible to this condition (perhaps through genetic predisposition or personal circumstances) find that their strong desire to obey the commandments of God can be translated into a preoccupation with rules of any kind.

Some illnesses take on a particular colouring for the Christian: the schizophrenic suffering from hallucinations may believe that the powers of evil are taking over his mind.

Even the Christian lifestyle may contribute to certain forms of breakdown. The leader who cannot refuse an invitation to speak or a call for a pastoral visit; the minister's wife who manages the home, the family and possibly a job as well as endless visitors and meetings; or the church member who drives himself too hard to meet impossibly high standards or work or study: all may end up suffering from overwork, burn-out or anxiety.

Jeff Lucas is a popular and well-known Christian speaker, and a minister of Timberline Church, Colorado. He was the main speaker at the Elim Bible Week at Prestatyn in 2004. There he revealed in public for the first time that he had suffered from clinical depression. In a recent edition of Direction magazine he said that in bringing depression out of the closet he had helped large numbers of people, "especially because the medical profession say that Christians can be the very worst at dealing with depression, refusing to take their medication, and being paralysed by an irrational guilt". He added, "If we broke our arm, we wouldn't hesitate to use a sling – but when our heads hurt, some of us feel that we should be able to deal with it without the assistance of medication." To the query, "How did you cope?" he replied, "I kept going. I talked to a few trusted friends. I took the tablets."

Confusions

The secular world tends to regard the human being as having two constituent parts – body and mind. Sometimes the view is even more limited, and the mind or personality is seen as merely a delusion, a trick played on us by the chemicals and electrical impulses in the brain, which is undeniably merely an organ in the physical body. Christians, however, add a third element: the spirit or soul.

Jesus had no difficulty with this. There are records in the Gospels of his healing touch in every aspect of people's lives: he healed those who were physically sick, he restored the mind of the deranged man and he forgave sins. Yet some Christians find it difficult to comprehend the fusion of body, mind and spirit that we believe constitutes wholeness. The psalmist says, "I praise you, for I am fearfully and wonderfully made" (Psalm 139:14). There is a complex overlap between the three elements of our being.

The body has in the past had a bad press – particularly in the church, which has often been condemnatory of the "sins of the flesh" as though these could happen without the will being implicated! I think it is always important to see the body as the temple of the Holy Spirit, the physical form into which God has breathed life, and respect it for that.

The mind is generally regarded as the seat of the personality – the part that is essentially the self. Psychology identifies three aspects of the function of the mind:

- cognition – the process of thinking, understanding and perception

- affect – mood, emotions and feelings

- conation – motivation, planning and the use of the will.

The elaborate interaction of these three functions enables us to think, learn, respond, act and construct meaningful relationships with other people.

If there are distortions in any of these functions, observable changes take place in our behaviour. For instance, our feelings are an important part of our personal life: our mood can be good or bad, and it varies from day to day, according to events and relationships. If our feelings are disordered for any length of time, we can fall prey to an illness such as depression, one of the most common conditions. The World Health Organisation has estimated that by 2020 it will be second only to heart disease as the biggest global health burden.[2] However, 40 per cent of those suffering with depression never consult their GPs.[3]

People increasingly understand that there are interactions between the body and the mind. There are somatoform disorders (sometimes called psychosomatic illnesses), where one's mental state causes physical symptoms, whether at the simplest level (such as a headache caused by stress) or the more complex (such as paralysis caused by mental trauma). Similarly, there may be psychiatric symptoms caused by physical illnesses (such as certain cases of depression which may be due to anaemia or cancer).

It is harder to define the spirit or the soul, yet Christians are convinced that it has as much objective reality as the other parts of what we call our "self". Some theology books have described it as the "psyche" as though it equated to the personality or even the mind. I am sure that it is more than that: it is the part of us that lives to eternity after our body dies; it is certainly not the same as mental capacity. Most of us know Christians whose intellectual abilities may be limited, but who demonstrate great spiritual awareness and strength.

One difficulty is that our perception of our spiritual life happens in our mind: we think about God; we have feelings about him, our fellow Christians and ourselves; and we can determine by our will to do God's will. These are the mental instruments of our spiritual life, and of course they are all involved when we suffer any spiritual disturbance. If we commit some sin, we think about it and use our understanding of the teaching of the Bible to identify it (cognition); we feel guilty about it, and after we have confessed it and been granted forgiveness we feel cleansed and happy (affect); we use our will to resolve not to fail in the same way in the future (conation).

Of course, just as we saw with the interaction between mind and body, the process can also work in reverse. If our thoughts and feelings are disturbed by an illness such as depression, it can have an effect on our spiritual life. I once knew a glorious Christian, a professional man known as a gracious leader, who suffered severe and recurrent depression. On those occasions he would come to my clinic, saying that he could no longer pray or read the Bible; it all seemed to him to be empty and meaningless. His condition was then exacerbated by his feelings of guilt that he could no longer reach out to God. That man needed treatment in both realms: medication for his depression and loving spiritual support. I would say to him, "Just hold on," and I would pray for him even when he could no longer find the words for himself. Once his depression lifted, he would once again be able to function spiritually, returning to scripture and to his prayer life with renewed enthusiasm.

Forsaken by God?

Many Christians become caught in a vicious circle of depression and guilt when mental illness is diagnosed. Often they see it as a form of weakness on their part, a failure and the measure of a faith that has been found lacking. In the major psychiatric illnesses, their depression can be so profound (and of delusional intensity) that they no longer believe they are accepted by God. Thinking that God has forsaken them is a very real and distressing condition to be in. We are reminded of Christ's anguish on the cross: "My God, my God, why have you forsaken me?" (Matthew 27:46). This passage itself can be a real comfort to Christians who find themselves in this situation. It shows how real and relevant the gospel is to our lives: Christ himself suffered from this feeling.

We should never belittle depression or fail to recognize its danger: 90 per cent of suicides result from depression, and there are around 6,000 suicides in the UK every year.[4] A proportion of these are Christians. It seems unthinkable that Christians should kill themselves, but they do, and when that happens in a church, a cloud falls upon it. Other church members feel guilty that they were unable to help, or that their pastoral care was inadequate. We can hardly bear to think of how distraught someone must be to arrive at the point of suicide. "He was out of his mind," people say, and in a sense they are right – the mind is not functioning properly when someone is suffering from depression.

Of course, the sufferer is never forsaken by God, no matter how much he or she may feel abandoned. God's grace is always extended to us, and he shows his love in many ways: through the loving support of family and friends, through the prayers and care of the church; and by the appropriate treatment available from the GP or the psychiatrist. The fact of spiritual grace does not in any way count against the proper treatment of mental illness: the two are not incompatible. If you have appendicitis, the appropriate treatment is an appendectomy. It is a simple operation, but it can be disastrous not to undergo it: peritonitis and death can result. The skill of the surgeon or the psychiatrist, and the efficacy of the antibiotic or the antidepressant are all God-given gifts from which we benefit. God has given us the knowledge and the medication to heal the sick, and it is only right that we accept help and thank him for it.

As a psychiatrist of many years' standing I deplore the stigma and fear that attach to mental illness, and that result in many people's reluctance to seek help. I have seen wonderful results from the proper treatment.

As a doctor (all psychiatrists are doctors who have completed their full medical training before going on to specialize in the treatment of mental illness) I advocate evidence-based medicine. That means appropriate treatments – whether through talking therapies or medication – which are proven to work and have delivered reproducible results. These treatments are available from the National Health Service and patients can trust them.

As a Christian, I also know that even after successful treatment, many people continue to feel unhappy, restless or unfulfilled, because their spiritual needs remain unmet. As early as the fourth century, St Augustine observed that humans have a "God-shaped space" inside them, and they can find peace only in an encounter with the living God. Those who feel unloved and alone can find joy and fulfilment in the companionship of the Holy Spirit. Those who suffer from feelings of inadequacy and guilt can find release in Jesus Christ, whose death wiped out their sins and who offers them new life.

There is hope for everyone who suffers from mental illness; fear, stigma and reluctance to seek help can all be reduced by better knowledge and understanding, which I hope this book will provide.

Notes

1 Source: The Mental Health Foundation.
2 World Health Report, *Noncommunicable Diseases and Mental Health* (World Health Organisation, May 2001).
3 *The Management of Depression in Primary and Secondary Care, Guideline No 23* (National Institute of Clinical Excellence).
4 Source: Office for National Statistics.

2

FACT OR FICTION?

Mental illness can be hard for the observer to understand. If someone breaks a leg, no one would expect them to sprint or even go for a brisk walk. Yet people who are suffering from depression are often told bracingly "Pull yourself together" or "Count your blessings," and encouraged to "Get out and meet people." This betrays a real ignorance of the nature of mental illness. The man with a broken leg has a plaster cast which everyone can see, and he receives sympathy and understanding. The sufferer from depression may have no visible sign of illness.

Many sufferers themselves say wonderingly, "I had everything – a good job, a nice home, a loving family. I had nothing to be depressed about." They cannot understand it themselves. Yet once depression – or anxiety, or a phobia – has taken hold, no one can expect sufferers to "snap out of it". They simply do not have sufficient control of their mental processes.

There are people who stubbornly refuse to believe that mental illnesses – or at least the more common neuroses – are real at all. (They are usually compelled to admit that the more severe psychotic states, involving delusions or hallucinations, are evidently illnesses.) These people sometimes believe that only conditions that require medication are "real". They observe that mild depression and other conditions can sometimes be improved or cured by "talking therapies", and they assume that such therapy

27

has no more scientific basis than a chat over a cup of tea with a friend. And if he can be cured by that, they think, surely the patient is suffering from an imaginary illness, no more severe than the passing low moods that we all experience. This view is wrong on several counts: the "talking therapies" require trained and skilled therapists; depression may begin with a low mood but it can increase dramatically in severity; and mental illness can be disabling mentally, socially and even physically.

Another reason why mental illness is hard to understand is that it is hard to define, and definitions themselves may be culturally conditioned. For instance, in Western society someone who is addicted to gambling is easily recognized as suffering from an obsession. Yet it is common to encounter people who spend their whole lives in the pursuit of wealth, and no one would dream of suggesting that these people are mad or suffering from a mental illness. They work incredibly long hours and take little or no leisure time; they sacrifice relationships with their families and friends; they have no hobbies or interests outside work; they buy land, large houses, fast cars and designer clothes, although they have little opportunity to enjoy any of their possessions. They constantly seek power, prestige, fame or even fashion to the point of obsession – yet this is regarded as normal behaviour in our society.

Similarly, there is evidence of an increase in alcoholism in the UK, with many young people not only binge drinking at weekends, but needing to drink every day; but most of these people would deny that they are suffering from alcohol dependency. It is their cultural norm to get drunk on most nights of the week. Recognizing certain illnesses depends on the local culture.

Some nationalities scarcely recognize mental illness at all. In South-east Asia post-traumatic stress disorder

(PTSD) is unknown; after the tsunami of 2004 many people complained of physical pains or sleeplessness, but seldom identified the probable cause. Sri Lanka did not even have a word for depression until one was coined in recent years.[1]

Identifying causes

There may be many causes for mental disturbance, and these are the subject of ongoing debate. One may be genetic predisposition: just as we inherit physical characteristics from our parents, so we may inherit personality types. Some people may be more likely to develop particular physical illnesses, such as cystic fibrosis or cancer, and others may be more susceptible to mental illnesses, such as schizophrenia. There is some evidence of a disposition to mental illnesses running in families.

Family background may also be a trigger: someone who grows up in particularly difficult circumstances, feeling insecure or afraid or being abused, may be more vulnerable to mental disturbance. Children who are discouraged from expressing their emotions may bottle up their feelings and suffer from the resulting stress.

People react in different ways to life events, such as bereavement, accident or illness. Traumatic events may cause long-term stress in some people, while others seem to manage them more easily. This is not an indicator of weakness or strength, merely of differences in personality and outlook. For instance, some depression after a bereavement is so common that it is regarded as part of the normal pattern of grieving.

The mind may also be affected by our body chemistry: for instance, experiencing excitement or danger triggers the body's "fight or flight" reaction, causing the release of a hormone called adrenalin. This stimulates the liver to release more glucose into the bloodstream, to be broken down for energy. It also stimulates an increase in the heart rate, faster breathing and blood vessel constriction. If this energy is not used up in physical activity, the body remains in a state of high alert and the mind over-active. Over a long period of such stress, depression and anxiety may result.

There may be other physical causes for mental illness. Certain acute conditions (that is, having a rapid onset) produce mental confusion, but they are often transient and the patient makes a full recovery. Such physical causes may include: infections in the brain; trauma such as head injuries; tumours (both benign and malignant); neurological conditions that affect the brain as well as the peripheral nerves; endocrine disorders that affect the brain; and other general systematic conditions of the heart and lungs, which can lead to anoxia (lack of oxygen) and affect the brain.

There are also chronic conditions, in which there is a steady progressive cognitive impairment resulting in dementia. These illnesses, such as Huntingdon's chorea and Pick's disease, generally occur in middle age and are termed pre-senile dementias. Creutzfeldt-Jakob disease (CJD) is a rare and fatal neurodegenerative disease that produces rapidly progressing dementia; patients are usually between the ages of fifty and seventy-five. However, in 1996 a new variant was reported, which seems to affect younger people; there is evidence that it is caused by bovine spongiform encephalopathy ("mad cow disease"). In spite of great anxiety at the time, which caused the removal of all beef products of a certain age from the food chain, there have been fewer cases than predicted and knowledge of the disease remains limited.

Mental health

In the absence of specific physical causes, there are things people can do to help themselves and improve their general mental health.

Relaxation is a useful skill – whether acquired from classes, tapes and CDs, or meditation and prayer. Physical activity can support both physical and mental well-being, raising a low mood and enhancing self-esteem. Learning to be assertive helps many people who suffer tension and anxiety because they find it hard to stand up for themselves. Similarly, learning to express feelings instead of repressing them can help people recover from hurtful experiences more easily. Facing up to problems instead of hiding from them, and setting goals to improve one's life are all recommended courses of action, but these are often hard to achieve alone. In such situations it is often helpful to find someone to talk to, whether this is a trusted friend, a church elder, leader or minister, a counsellor or a therapist, or a self-help or support group.

These suggestions come from MIND, the mental health organization, as a range of activities which may be helpful to everyone, whether they suffer from mental illness or not. This adds another element of confusion to the "Fact or Fiction?" debate. If mental health can be improved in these simple ways, asks the doubter, how can mental disturbance be regarded as an illness? Surely these proven aids amount to no more than the despised advice to "pull yourself together".

In fact, they make sense because of the links between body and mind (hence the fact that physical exercise is a well-known mood enhancer) and also between the brain (the physical organ, affected by chemical changes), the mind (the perception of our consciousness and personality) and our behaviour (the way in which our mental condition is expressed). It is because of these links that some conditions such as mild depression, anxiety and phobias, can be treated by "talking therapies", which affect our patterns of thought and behaviour, and others can be better treated by medication that returns the brain chemistry to normal. There is overlap between these conditions, and either or both treatments may be appropriate.

Crossing boundaries

There is no doubt that some mental illnesses are "spectrum" conditions – that is, they range from the very mild to very severe. At the mild end of the spectrum, symptoms may be considered to be so common as to be evidence of normality; for instance, it is usual to feel some anxiety about certain activities (such as hang-gliding, mountain climbing or other extreme sports – that is their attraction). It is only if this anxiety becomes severe and inappropriately attached to everyday activities, such as leaving the house, that it would be considered as a mental illness.

When symptoms amount to merely an exaggeration of normal traits, sufferers may persist in seeing them as normal and do not recognize that they have crossed a boundary from mental health to illness. Some anxiety is normal: if you did not suffer from any anxiety at all, you would be suffering from something worse, because only psychopaths have no feelings. That anxiety fluctuates in intensity, depending on our circumstances and the stresses in our lives. It is only when anxiety is no longer controllable, and does not respond to reassurance, that it becomes an illness.

At the point of crossing that boundary, physiological

changes may be observed: the heart rate increases, the patient sweats and may even experience chest pains. The general state of anxiety may become focused on one particular object. Once that boundary has been crossed, it is impossible for the patient to "pull himself together".

This is where we can explore the blurred boundary between "neurotic" and "psychotic" states. The usual way of explaining these is to say that a neurosis causes the sufferer very real distress, but the patient retains insight, self-awareness and contact with reality. He may be unable to help himself but he knows that he is worrying unnecessarily. Psychosis is more severe in that the patient loses insight and becomes divorced from reality: it is a symptom of the major illnesses such as severe depression, schizophrenia and paranoid states.

The neuroses are often regarded as the milder forms of mental and emotional illnesses, although even neurotic symptoms can be so severe that they paralyze a person's life. A woman suffering from agoraphobia may be so socially impaired that she is unable to go out to shop or take her children to school; she may become a prisoner in her own home.

The psychoses are characterized by the loss of insight: patients complain of hallucinations (sensations without adequate stimulus) and delusions (false beliefs, impervious to reason). For instance, patients may suffer from the paranoid delusion that someone is poisoning their food, or conspiring against them, when this has no basis in fact and there is no evidence for this at all. However much friends and doctors try to explain and reassure the patients, they insist that what they believe is true. Church members will often have met with certain forms of paranoia: the person in church who is always worried about being slighted or left out of things, who complains that others are giving them strange looks or talking about them behind their back. The difficulty is knowing when these mild personality traits of suspicion and low self-esteem cross the boundary into a paranoid psychosis.

Offering hope

It is often the case that a diagnosis of mental illness is not rejected; rather, the sufferer welcomes it with open arms. This is not because the patient is perverse and wishes to be ill; rather, it is often because they have been feeling so bad that they feared that they were going mad. Someone who is suffering from depression may come to the doctor because they have a range of physical symptoms, from exhaustion to headaches. They may fear a diagnosis of cancer; equally, they fear being told that there is nothing wrong with them and that therefore nothing can be done to make them feel better. They may even have already been told by family and friends to "pull themselves together" – something they are certainly incapable of doing. If that were possible, they would have done so already: they do not wish to go on feeling like this.

So the diagnosis confirms that they really are ill. They have an illness with a name, with readily identifiable symptoms, which other people have suffered from. They are not alone; they are not going mad. In short, they have the doctor's permission to be ill. Paradoxically, this in itself can make people feel considerably better.

I was once consulted by the mother of a child who had cerebral palsy. Mrs Brown did not come to see me initially for herself: she actually needed a medical legal report, which I could provide, on behalf of her daughter. However, it rapidly became clear to me that she herself, worn out with caring for her disabled daughter, was actually suffering from depression.

We spent some time discussing her problems and difficulties, and I explained that as a psychiatrist I was able make to such a diagnosis. I explained about the nature of depression, and she was astounded that I was able to describe her symptoms so accurately. I was then able to tell her that there was treatment available for her, and that the antidepressants I was prescribing would make her feel better very quickly.

When she left my office, before she had even obtained her prescription, let alone taken a tablet, she said to me, "Healing began for me today." When I asked her what she meant, she said, "You are the only doctor who has ever asked me how I felt. You have given me hope, and I shall live." It was the diagnosis and the promise of treatment which gave her comfort and the hope of healing, things that were very important to her.

Mrs Brown was a Christian, and I knew that the words of Psalm 40 would be appropriate for her:

> *I waited patiently for the Lord;*
>   *he inclined to me and heard my cry.*
> *He drew me up from the desolate pit,*
>   *out of the miry bog,*
> *and set my feet upon a rock,*
>   *making my steps secure.*
> *He put a new song of praise into my mouth,*
>   *a song of praise to our God.*
>
> Psalm 40:2–3

Once we have accepted that mental illness is a fact of life, it is useful to increase our knowledge of the various kinds of illnesses and the treatments available.

Notes

1 Dr Palitha Abeykoon, who works on mental health issues for the
  World Health Organization, quoted in the *New York Times*, 24
  January 2005.

3

MENTAL ILLNESSES

We have seen how difficult it is to understand mental illness, and to define the boundaries between mental health and illness, and between one illness and another. Many symptoms are common to several different conditions, so that precise diagnosis can be difficult. In addition, some of the terms (such as depression, anxiety and panic) are used in a non-clinical sense in ordinary conversation, causing further confusion to the layperson who wonders what exactly constitutes a mental illness.

Alcohol and drug dependence

These conditions may be both physical and psychological, resulting from the response of the body to the substance – the "high" experienced when using alcohol or the drug. With repeated use, tolerance may develop, so the user has to take larger amounts to achieve the same effect. Not taking the substance may lead to uncomfortable or painful withdrawal symptoms, both physical and psychological.

Once someone has become dependent on drink or drugs, both physical and mental health may suffer, with consequent effects on personal relationships and the ability to work. This may cause other problems such as unemployment, poverty, isolation and homelessness.

Drug misuse may include illegal drugs such as cannabis, LSD, heroin or cocaine, or excessive use of medication available from doctors on prescription. Alcohol, which is both legal and readily available, is an increasing problem: 27 per cent of men and 15 per cent of women regularly drink more than the recommended limit.[1]

When people wish to end their substance misuse, a combination of physical and psychological treatments may be necessary. Doctors can prescribe other drugs (usually in decreasing amounts) to relieve the withdrawal symptoms; this may be offered in specialist drug or alcohol units, either in outpatients' departments or residential institutions. Dealing with the psychological dependence on drugs or alcohol usually requires support, either through "talking treatments" (psychotherapy) or counselling support from such organisations as Alcoholics Anonymous or Narcotics Anonymous.

Anxiety

Anxiety is an emotional state characterised by apprehension, uncertainty, dread or fear: it may be defined as a state of anticipation of something unpleasant about to happen. It occurs in normal situations and has positive aspects: it can be a defence against engaging in dangerous activities, or provide the energy that enables us to take on a challenge. Everyone is familiar with the dry mouth, racing heart and sweaty palms that may accompany a job interview or an important exam: the adrenalin makes us extra alert and able to acquit ourselves well. It is only when the "nerves" take over that our anxiety becomes disabling, so that the actor ceases to be merely keyed up for his performance, but is prevented from performing at all because of stage fright.

When anxiety becomes constant and unrealistic, it has crossed the boundary into mental illness. It may be an undirected emotional state (termed "free-floating" anxiety), or it may become focused on a particular object (when it is usually known as a phobic state). Some 4 or 5 per cent of adults experience generalized anxiety disorders that do not include depression at any one time.[2] A further 9 per cent have mixed anxiety and depression; this is more common in women than men.

Anxiety neurosis has symptoms of both a physical and psychological nature. The physical symptoms can affect most of the body: muscles become tense and the patient suffers from tightness of the chest, sweating, palpitations, dry mouth, pallor, feelings of cold, gastric discomfort, choking sensations and trembling. All these symptoms indicate that the psychological state has affected the autonomic nervous system, producing very real physical sensations.

Patients suffering from an anxiety neurosis often worry about their physical state. Sleep patterns may show marked disturbances, often insomnia in which the patient has difficulty falling asleep. In addition there will be general restlessness and unease, problems with concentration and occasionally defective memory, though this is seldom true amnesia. (Compare the student whose mind goes blank when he sits in front of an examination paper; half an hour after the examination ends, he can recall clearly all the facts that eluded him earlier.)

The worrying thoughts become repetitive, to the extent that patients often think they are going mad; they fear that they are having a breakdown, and feel guilty that they are unable to cope with ordinary life. Christians are particularly prone to these feelings of guilt. They know that the Lord Jesus Christ promised them peace: "Peace I leave with you; my peace I give to you. I do not give to you as the world gives. Do not let your hearts be troubled, and do not let them be afraid" (John 14:27). They feel that they are failing him when they are consumed with worry and anxiety.

This condition may be a mild mental illness, yet it affects patients' behaviour, personality, interpersonal relationships and indeed the whole of their life. They retain the insight that allows them to see reality, and understand that it is "silly to feel so anxious" when there is no stress in their lives to cause such a level of anxiety. Nevertheless they are unable to shake off their fears, and the "pull yourself together" advice is quite useless. This is just what they cannot do. It is similarly useless to quote biblical advice to Christians, as they often end up feeling even more guilty for the failure of their faith. It is imperative that they accept that they are suffering from a real illness, realize its significance and are prepared to accept the appropriate therapy. They are no less of a Christian for suffering in this way, and should not feel guilty if they are referred for treatment to a psychiatrist or another therapist.

Panic attacks

Panic attacks are sudden, unexpected episodes of intense terror, when the anxiety becomes extremely focused and severe. Many of the symptoms of anxiety are present – increased heart rate, difficulty in breathing, choking sensations or pains in the chest, accompanied by shaking or faintness. Sufferers may even mistake the symptoms for a heart attack or other illness. They can happen at any time, but if the sufferer experiences a panic attack in a particular place (e.g. in a crowded shop) he or she may begin to avoid that situation in an attempt to prevent a recurrence.

Around seven people in a thousand develop a panic disorder, and this figure is roughly the same for men and women and across all age groups.[3]

Phobic states

Phobic anxiety disorders have the same core systems as the generalized anxiety already described, but they tend to occur in particular and predictable circumstances. As a result, patients try to avoid the circumstances that provoke them, and they experience anticipatory anxiety when there is a possibility of encountering such situations. The triggers for anxiety may be objects (such as spiders), situations (such as crowded rooms) or natural phenomena (such as thunder) – the patient may begin to feel anxious at the first sign of a storm, or at the suggestion that they attend a meeting. It is usual to recognize three principal phobic states: the simple, the social and agoraphobia.

Simple phobias are usually of objects or situations, and are very common. Many people are happy to admit to a fear of snakes or spiders, of flying, of being in high places such as tall buildings or cliff tops, or enclosed spaces (claustrophobia).

Patients suffering from social phobia become inappropriately anxious in situations in which they are observed and could be criticized, so they tend to avoid being in groups, taking part in conversation or speaking in public. These feelings usually stem from deep-rooted feelings of inadequacy, and are subconscious – a part of the personality. Occasionally these people respond to being in company with others by exhibiting excited speech and aggressive behaviour.

People suffering from agoraphobia are anxious when away from home, in crowds or in situations or places from which they cannot easily escape. These may include buses, shops, trains and supermarkets. They develop anxiety symptoms, including anxious thoughts about panic attacks, fainting and loss of control, and display anticipatory anxiety, often hours before the event.

There is another kind of agoraphobia that begins in the mid twenties or early thirties. It arises from conscious but unacceptable sexually aggressive urges, or occasionally a tendency to fear minor physical symptoms; there seems to be a failure of the brain mechanisms that control anxiety.

These conditions usually need referral to a specialist therapist: a general counsellor can give support and encourage a staged return to the situations that arouse anxiety, avoiding the condition becoming chronic. These phobias can be successfully treated by behaviour therapy, which includes exposure to the stimulant and training to cope with panic attacks.

Dementia

Dementia is largely an illness of the elderly: it affects 6 per cent of people between sixty-five and eighty, but 20 per cent of those over eighty. Over two-thirds of these are diagnosed with Alzheimer's Disease.[4] The major symptoms are loss of recent memory, poor comprehension, emotional instability and a tendency to self-neglect. It is caused by physical changes to the brain.

Hysterical states

Hysterical neurosis is a disorder characterised by mental dissociation; it often leads to somatic (physical) symptoms such as convulsions, fits, paralysis and sensory disturbances, though there is no organic disease. In other cases it can lead to multiple personality and amnesia. Often the illness is employed for some secondary gain, though the patient is not fully aware of this motive.

Hysterics can cause a great deal of difficulty in any group, including the church. Their narcissistic and immature behaviour demands attention from the minister, elders and other members, and they can be manipulative, refusing to respond unless they get their own way. It is important to be able to recognize and diagnose the condition within a fellowship, but there are many problems. Some individuals are exhibiting personality disorders with these marked narcissistic traits; others suffer from a complete hysterical neurosis. It is hard to tell how far the suffering is genuine or feigned; how much is wilful action and how much unconscious neurosis.

Obsessional responses to stress and anxiety suggest a desire for rigid control; hysterical symptoms, on the contrary, seem to be due to loss of control, producing some startling symptoms and behaviour.

There are two kinds of hysterical states: conversion disorders and dissociative disorders. In the first, an anxiety may be removed from the awareness and converted into physical symptoms. For instance, a young mother presented with a loss of power in her right arm, which eventually became entirely paralyzed. No physical cause could be found for this, but deep counselling revealed an unconscious aggression towards her second child. Her arm had become paralysed as a defence against hurting the child. Hers was a true illness: she was completely unaware of the difficulty in her subconscious mind.

In the second kind of hysterical state, the awareness may become split up by a process of dissociation of consciousness. This is manifested mainly as psychological conditions such as amnesia and multiple personalities. The fictional account of *Dr Jekyll and Mr Hyde*, in Robert Louis Stevenson's story, is a classic example. However, such dissociative states occur commonly in real life. A man who was under great stress at home and in business was found 200 miles away from home, unable to remember his identity. It was several weeks before he recovered his memory.

When the dissociation is very severe it can occur as multiple personalities. At the beginning of the last century there was a very famous case of a woman who apparently had three distinct personalities, which was described in the book *The Three Faces of Eve*.[5]

It is important that these conditions are understood in religious circles, because we know that these psychological manifestations can occur in the course of magical religious rites. These seem to arise from unconscious mechanisms rather than from conscious stimulation. There are also undoubtedly forms of possession in religious experience that are examples of hysterical dissociation, such aswhen the person is in a state of trance, assuming a different voice and character. Similar states can occur in psychotic disorders such as schizophrenia. This is why it is so important that Christian leaders take care when diagnosing so-called "possession" states, and that they understand the underlying condition.

While the remedies for hysterical states will be dealt with in the section on treatment, it is useful to note that for acute hysterical conditions (especially on their first occurrence), reassurance and suggestion are usually an appropriate and adequate response. This must, of course, be supported by the sufferer's own determination to resolve the problem that precipitated the attack. Symptoms lasting more than a few weeks need to be referred to a specialist; by then it is much harder to treat the case because the unconscious conflict causes a block between the mind and the body.

It is essential that patients who present with physical manifestations of a conversion disorder get the offer of an honourable retreat and an excuse to get better, by recognizing their problems and being helped to alleviate them. One of my patients used to return to the outpatients' clinic every summer with a so-called "paralysis of the legs". The first time I saw him I realized that he was suffering a hysterical reaction to his ogre of a mother, who demanded too much of him emotionally and physically. One of his responsibilities every summer was to "do the garden", a huge plot of land. His paralysis was a way out of facing this hard work. His mother used to attend the clinic with him and reinforced his difficulties. I was able to tell her and his friends to encourage him to walk, and he found he was able to do so. He accepted that we were aware of his difficulties, that he was suffering from hysteria and that he was able to deal with the basic problem. Unfortunately he still had to return to his gardening. One almost sympathized with his hysterical reaction.

Malingering

In dealing with such hysterical symptoms we must face the question of how to differentiate between hysteria, other neuroses and malingering. Often the layperson will think that someone whose symptoms have no physical cause is "putting it on", that he wills to do it and is therefore malingering. There is an important difference: the malingerer is consciously manipulating the situation and is fully aware of his actions; the hysteric is quite unaware of the mental cause of his very real physical symptoms.

Whereas hysterical neurosis with its unconscious motivation is an illness, malingering is not. A malingerer is a person presenting with physical or psychological symptomology, deliberately setting out to deceive for his own gain, often to avoid work, to bring a civil action (e.g. suing an organization for causing stress or an accident) or to defraud an insurance company. This can amount to a criminal act which may be prosecuted. Therefore people such as Christian leaders, lawyers, doctors, social workers, employers and anyone who has occasion to deal with such conditions must be particularly careful about such labels and how they use them.

Obsessive-compulsive disorder

When anxiety cannot be controlled it may result in Obsessive-compulsive disorder (OCD): around 1 per cent of the population suffer from this at any one time.[6] Obsessional neurosis is characterized by the persistent obtrusion into the consciousness of ideas or emotional states, obsessions or compulsive impulses to action. This happens independently of the patient's will, without a cause that is evident to their consciousness, and in spite of the fact that they are able to recognize its irrational character. It is striking that many Christians suffer from OCD.

After my book *Healing the Hurt Mind* was published in 1983, I was contacted by a young Christian man who lived in Australia. He had suffered for years from paralysing guilt because of his secret obsessive-compulsive symptoms. In spite of therapy and counselling he had found no adequate explanation for his symptoms, and they had persisted to a significant degree. When he read the chapter on obsessional states he finally felt that someone understood him; once he himself understood that he was suffering from a recognized mental illness his guilt was assuaged, and he was so excited by this that he telephoned the author at three o'clock in the morning!

The symptoms are readily identifiable and they cause great tension within the individual. The outstanding feature is the feeling of subjective compulsion, which initially the victim tries to resist, to carry out some action or to dwell on a specific thought or idea. These unwanted thoughts intrude unprovoked, and the victim sees them as inappropriate or nonsensical. The obsessional urge or idea is recognized as alien to the personality, but also as coming from within themselves.

Christians are often particularly perturbed by these compulsions because they feel that they are being controlled by a force outside themselves, which they immediately assume to be evil. Often their obsessional thoughts have sexual connotations and may be pornographic, and the victims thus feel "dirty" and unworthy of their Christian calling, adding to their guilt. Christian friends may suggest that these thoughts are demonic, adding to the sufferer's fear and misery.

A Christian man in late middle age, who had a good job and a loving family, suffered greatly because of what he called "dirty" thoughts that came into his mind. Sexual thoughts would enter his consciousness when he was trying to read his Bible, and nothing he could do would prevent their intrusion. This caused him tremendous suffering and he often despaired. Some Christians in whom he had confided had suggested that the devil was the cause of his trouble, because the thoughts seemed to come from outside him, and this made him feel even more guilty. It was only after treatment that he gained insight into his condition and understood that these were common neurotic symptoms; after specific therapy he improved and his guilt cleared.

Obsessions

Obsessions are repeated thoughts or actions that enter the consciousness of the sufferer. All attempts to dispel these unwelcome urges lead only to a more severe inner struggle, and tension increases until the victim "gives in" and allows the thoughts to intrude or reverts to a repetition of the action. Relief is only temporary and the urge builds up again, until a vicious circle is established.

• Obsessional thoughts consist of single words, phrases or rhymes which are usually unpleasant or shocking to the victim.

• Obsessional imagery involves imagined scenes, often of a violent or disgusting kind, which may include certain sexual practices.

• Obsessional ruminations are internal diatribes in which arguments for and against even the simplest everyday actions are reviewed continually.

• Obsessional doubts concern actions that may or may not have been completed adequately (such as turning off the gas taps or locking the door); others may concern actions that may have harmed other people, or fear that they may do so in the future. Sometimes doubts are related to religious convictions and observances, and these can cause particular stress to Christians.

• Obsessional impulses are urges to perform acts, usually of a violent or embarrassing nature, such as leaping in front of a car, injuring a child or shouting out in church. Again, the Christian is particularly threatened by this kind of symptom. The young Martin Luther suffered from this condition, and experienced the urge to blaspheme in the sanctuary of the church.

• Obsessional rituals include mental activities (such as counting in a special way or repeating a certain form of words) and also behaviours (such as washing the hands twenty or even a hundred times a day).

It is not difficult to understand how paralyzing this kind of condition is. Even though it is a neurosis and the patient retains insight into the unreasonableness of the behaviour, the suffering is great and the effect on a person's life is immense. The ritual behaviours in particular can dominate a person's life. Some have understandable connections with obsessional thoughts that precede them, such as repeated washings after touching something dirty. Other rituals have no specific connection, such as laying out clothes in a complicated but set pattern before dressing. Some patients are compelled to repeat such actions a certain number of times, and if something goes wrong with the process they have to start the whole sequence over again.

Patients are invariably aware that their rituals are illogical and they try to hide them. Some feel that these symptoms are a sign that they are going mad, and they can be greatly helped by reassurance that this is not so. However, the condition still causes great distress to them and to other family members. Partners may begin to feel increasingly irritated by the compulsions. Tension within the family can be reduced by counselling and reassurance: feelings of unease and anger are perfectly normal when attempting to live with these difficult behaviours.

Eating disorders

Anorexia nervosa presents as a distorted attitude to self-image, with particular reference to body weight: sufferers commonly believe that they are "too fat" (even though they may actually be underweight), and deliberately restrict their eating in the hope of slimming. They often try to hide their condition, secretly disposing of food. In the case of bulimia nervosa there may be episodes of "binge eating", followed by vomiting and excessive use of laxatives. This condition often takes a fluctuating course over several years and may leave long-lasting abnormal eating habits. In severe cases the fasting may be so extreme that it endangers life.

Up to 1 per cent of women in the UK between the ages of fifteen and thirty suffer from anorexia nervosa, and between 1 and 2 per cent from bulimia nervosa.[7] It may be that the actual figures are higher than this, as many cases of eating disorder likely to be unreported or undiagnosed. Eating disorders occur more commonly among women than men.

Prognosis for OCD

Occasionally the tension associated with these compulsions and obsessions can be so severe that it is possible to term them "obsessional psychosis". The intensity of the compulsions is so strong that they cannot be resisted or reduced. However, it is helpful to note that those with OCD do not go on to develop schizophrenia or other psychotic conditions, although they may develop depressive disorders.

Around two-thirds of all cases improve within one year. Cases lasting longer than a year usually take a fluctuating course, with periods of partial or complete remission lasting for months or several years. Severe cases may be exceedingly persistent but generally the prognosis is good, which is comforting for patients and their families. Victims should be reassured that they are not going mad and there is every chance that their symptoms will remit within a year.

It is particularly important to reassure Christians that the source of their thoughts, even when blasphemous, is not demonic.

Relatives often ask about the best way to deal with obsessive patients, as they themselves share in the inconvenience and distress of this condition. They should be included in discussions of the case (with the agreement of the patient, who is usually helped by this sharing). They can be shown how to be firm but compassionate, reminding the sufferer that there is hope of a definite improvement in the future.

Post-traumatic stress disorder

In recent years many emotional disorders related to stress have come to the fore. Some of these are minor conditions in which people complain of being worried, despondent or sad; often there is a mixture of such symptoms which do not quite fit any pattern. Some people will complain of some physical concern, and some will be mainly preoccupied with their physical symptoms. Many have difficulty sleeping because of obsessional thoughts.

One outstanding such disorder is post-traumatic stress disorder (PTSD). This appears to have become more common recently, perhaps because there has been an increasing amount of litigation associated with it. The condition is classically diagnosed when it follows a massive stressful event which would cause any normal person distress – usually involving a direct threat to life, or a situation in which the person believed he would be killed. This entry criterion must be met if a person is to be diagnosed as suffering from the condition. In addition, there will be one or more cardinal symptoms of reliving the event (such as flashbacks), intrusive thoughts that enter the consciousness quite unprovoked, and avoidance (where the person will try to avoid seeing the site of the event or even speaking about it). The person will also exhibit an active avoidance of any circumstances resembling or associated with the stressor (such as travelling by tube or any public transport after a bomb blast in the underground), which was not present before the event. There will be symptoms of increased psychological sensitivity and arousal such as difficulty in falling or staying asleep, irritability or outbursts of anger, difficulty in concentrating, hyper-vigilance and exaggerated startled response.

Many people have suffered from post-traumatic stress disorder after events such as the Lockerbie plane crash, the fire at King's Cross underground station, train crashes, the London terrorist attacks and other local disasters such as floods or fires. Other forms of post-traumatic stress disorder have been diagnosed after road traffic accidents and more minor stressful events. Some psychiatrists have suggested that this is a dubious diagnosis which owes more to the modern litigation culture than to good psychiatric practice: there is a tendency to blame other people for any mishap, and to try to get some compensation for it.

Schizophrenia

Schizophrenia is one of a group of important mental illnesses that vary fundamentally from those described above. The conditions already described are neurotic illnesses in which, however severe they are, the person maintains insight and remains in touch with reality. Schizophrenia and some other mental illnesses are known as psychotic disorders, and the common feature is that patients lack insight and are divorced from reality.

Schizophrenia is a relatively common illness among young people: around one in a hundred people will suffer from it at some time in their life (about the same as manic depression).[8] The symptoms generally appear between the ages of sixteen and twenty-two, and the condition is twice as common among males. Surprisingly, there is no evidence of any definitive macroscopic brain damage and no clear-cut reproducible neurobiochemical disorder. More surprisingly, even with the recent development of new brain-imaging techniques, we still have not found one definitive causal factor, though studies do indicate some changes in cerebral structure and function.

Many doctors believe that schizophrenia results from an interaction of genetic predisposition and environmental factors. There is strong evidence that schizophrenia has important genetic causes, although the mode of inheritance is not yet known.[9] Neurodevelopmental factors, such as cognitive and social impairment in childhood, and current stressful life events often provoke the disorder. Drugs such as cannabis and LSD can precipitate an acute schizophrenic episode.

Major symptoms are:

• Incongruity of mood – the patient may be thinking sad thoughts but may be laughing at the same time.

• Introversion and autism – where the patient withdraws from the world around him. He will be reluctant to talk and friends and family find it difficult to communicate with him.

• Disordered thought – speech will be irrelevant and nonsensical, even making up words and phrases not used in normal language. This is evidence of the degree of disintegration of normal thought patterns.

• False beliefs and delusions – patients may believe that people are plotting against them, or that their families are trying to poison them.

• Hallucinations – these may be either visual or auditory. Patients often say that they hear voices from outside their head when there is no one else present. These voices seem to read their thoughts and describe what they are thinking, and talk in a critical manner about them.

Like some forms of mania, schizophrenia can lead to ecstasy states where there will be some religious or philosophical material. This has sometimes been called "religious mania", suggesting that it is caused by religion. This is a fallacy; there can be conditions where religious references colour the thought, but no mania is caused by religion.

It is important to be aware of the implications. I once had a patient from a religious family who announced that he had experienced a religious conversion. He became preoccupied with reading the scriptures and prayer, but his behaviour became so extreme and bizarre that his family were forced to consider the possibility that he was ill. I examined him and was forced to diagnose a schizophrenic illness. His parents were very sad to hear this, but understood that what their son required was proper treatment.

I also met a non-Christian family who were similarly very disturbed when their daughter joined a religious group and announced that she had been "saved". She, too began to read the Bible and pray, and her lifestyle changed completely. Her parents feared that this was a schizophrenic illness and brought her for examination. I took a complete history from both parents and daughter and it became obvious that there was no evidence whatever of schizophrenia or any other mental illness. She was a very normal girl who had experienced a sudden, clear-cut religious conversion. Her parents were reassured and accepted the fact of her new lifestyle and beliefs.

Other psychotic conditions

Psychotic conditions share the core symptoms of delusions and/or hallucinations. A delusion is a false belief impervious to reason (bearing in mind the cultural background). During case management sessions I have witnessed certain members of the team trying to reason with a patient and trying to convince him that his belief was false, but failing miserably. It is a waste of time to try to explain away a false belief. A hallucination (auditory or visual) is a perception experienced in the absence of an adequate external stimulus. (However, we know that hallucinations can also occur in normal people.)

Other psychotic conditions associated with schizophrenia include paranoid states, which range from ideas that one is being "done down" or put upon, to deep convictions of persecution; they are characterized by systematised delusions and hallucinations. Psychotic states are also associated with affective states (mood disorders). Indeed, severe depressive disorders may include delusions regarding the body and even the patient's financial status. Mania is also a psychotic condition and a mood disorder; it is characterized by hyperactivity and an excited, agitated mood. It is often observed as one phase of manic depression, or bipolar disorder.

Depression

Although depression is indeed a mental illness like others listed here, it is so common and so complex a condition that it seems right to give it an entire chapter of its own.

Notes

1 Source: Office for National Statistics, *General Household Survey* (1998).

2 Source: Office for National Statistics, quoted in MIND factsheet.

3 Source: Office for National Statistics, quoted in MIND factsheet.

4 *Assessing older people with dementia living in the community: practice issues for social and health services* (Social Services Inspectorate, 1996), quoted in MIND factsheet.

5 Corbett H. Thigpen and Hervey M. Checkley, *The Three Faces of Eve* (London: Secker & Warburg, 1957).

6 Source: Office for National Statistics, quoted in MIND factsheet.

7 Source: The Mental Health Foundation.

8 Source: The Mental Health Foundation.

9 P. McGuffin and R. Murray (eds), *The New Genetics of Mental Illness* (Oxford: Butterworth Heinemann, 1991).

4

DEPRESSION

Different people mean different things when they talk about depression; in ordinary conversation it may mean nothing more than a passing feeling of sadness. The word "depression" is certainly to do with mood or affect, and can be used to describe the feeling of low spirits, to various degrees. It may be entirely appropriate that we feel depressed because some event has caused us to be so, such as bereavement, disappointment, divorce or relationship difficulties. However, depressive neurosis and more severe conditions can have far-reaching effects on the sufferer.

Depression is a major illness in the United Kingdom: an estimated one in twenty people will have serious or "clinical" depression at any one time. Overall, depression affects around 10 per cent of the population.[1] Estimates of the lifetime prevalence of depression vary, ranging from one in six to one in four.[2] It can occur at any age but is most common in people aged twenty-five to forty-four years.[3] An estimated 15 per cent of people over sixty-five have depression, and an estimated 5 per cent have severe depression.[4] There is a correlation between depression in older people and living alone.[5] Older people living in residential care are significantly more likely to develop depression than those living in the community.[6] According to the World Health Organisation, by 2020 depressive disorder will be the second most important illness in the world (after cardiac disease).

Physical causes

Depression is the major symptom of depressive illness, but it can also be a symptom (along with anxiety) of other organic diseases. That is why it is important to understand that all psychiatrists are doctors, with the requisite medical training to conduct a proper examination to make certain that there is no organic basis for the illness. It is only when a general practitioner or consultant physician in psychological medicine has completed the necessary investigations that the patient will be diagnosed as suffering from a functional (not organic) illness or depression.

The importance of doing this preliminary physical examination cannot be over-emphasized. I have had a number of patients referred to me initially as depressives, in whom I have subsequently diagnosed various physical illnesses. I once saw a doctor who began to suffer from depression in middle age. He had been seen by a number of other doctors who could find no physical cause for his illness, and he was referred to me as suffering from severe depression. He was very depressed, withdrawn, lacking in energy, lethargic and complaining of weight loss and feelings of helplessness. I felt it was imperative that he was examined and X-rayed and that blood tests should be taken. He was found to have lung cancer, and his depression was secondary to this.

Another sixty-year-old woman was referred to me as a depressive. She complained of being low-spirited, unable to sleep, lethargic, and having lost her faith and the joy of living. On examination she was found to be suffering from hypothyroidism (thyroid disease); she needed treatment with the appropriate medication (thyroxine).

A young married woman with three children was referred as having post-natal depression – a reasonable assumption, as she had given birth to her third child six months previously. She, too, was depressed, lethargic, unable to cope, unable to pray, and felt that life was "too much" for her. On investigation she was found to be severely anaemic.

In all these cases it was vital to carry out a proper examination, and to treat the physical conditions with the appropriate medication. Although the first man's cancer proved to be terminal, in the other two cases the physical treatments were highly successful, and the depression disappeared as their physical condition improved.

Severe depression

Depressive disorder can occur without any physical lesion: it is a psychological condition, albeit with physical as well as psychological symptoms. Most severe episodes of depression last between three and nine months, although there is a high risk of recurrence.

One form of severe and frequently recurrent depression is manic depression: this involves extreme mood swings from depression to elation and over-activity. It is sometimes referred to as bipolar mood disorder to reflect the two mood states. Approximately one in a hundred adults in the United Kingdom will experience manic depression at some point in their lives.[7]

One of the risks of severe depression is suicide. Estimates show that 90 per cent of the people who commit suicide have been suffering from depression; suicide accounts for 20 per cent of all deaths of young people.[8] Some 75 per cent of all suicides are men (especially younger men);[9] between 1971 and 1998, the suicide rate for women in England and Wales almost halved, while in the same period the rate for men almost doubled.[10] The figures are alarming: in 2001 there were 5,910 suicides in the United Kingdom, equating to approximately one suicide every ninety minutes.[11]

Symptoms

It is the role of the psychiatrist to diagnose and try to assess the severity of the depressive disorder, before deciding on the appropriate course of treatment. (It is worth noting in passing that medication can be prescribed only by doctors such as GPs and specialists such as consultant psychiatrists. Clinical psychologists cannot prescribe antidepressants, and neither can nurses, though there are moves to allow some of the latter, along with pharmacists, to prescribe under certain conditions.) With improved teaching and training for all doctors in the area of psychiatry there has been an improvement in the diagnosis of depression in general practice.

Severe depressive illness may consist of a primary depressive disorder or the depressive element of a manic depressive psychosis; it can be distinguished by some or all of a range of symptoms. Whatever the classification used, the following constellation of symptoms are of the utmost importance in diagnosing a major depressive disorder.

• Central depressive mood – when the patient feels very low-spirited and miserable and nothing raises their spirits. Associated may be "anhedonia" – a lack of the joy of living.

• Lack of interest, reduced energy, marked tiredness and pessimistic thinking. Often the patient's appearance will be one of untidiness if not actual neglect.

• Feelings of helplessness and hopelessness; feeling

dejected and despairing. Often there is a paradox in the fact that the patient may have a good job, a good salary and be effective in his work, yet he will feel that he is doing badly and has no future.

The following are regarded as biological symptoms, which are of particular importance.

• Diurnal variation of the depressive mood. Generally the depression is worse in the mornings and improves slightly as the day goes on. This diurnal variation is very indicative, and patients often notice this particularly and volunteer the information to the doctor.

• Sleep disorders – there is usually persistent early-morning waking, and sleep is generally disturbed.

• Weight loss for no apparent reason – though often the appetite is poor.

• Loss of libido – and among women, amenorrhoea (no menstrual periods).

Other symptoms include:

• Guilt – patients believe that they are the cause of other people's troubles or the ills of the world.

• Suicidal thoughts – though generally patients are reluctant to talk about this. However, it is essential that doctors and therapists ask relevant questions. If patients admit to thinking about committing suicide, and that they have made definite plans for how, when and where they would do it, their responses should be taken very seriously indeed.

• Possible delusions – patients believe that they are living in poverty when they are quite well off, that they are ineffective at work when they are very conscientious. They may even believe that they are "rotting away" or even dead. There may be hallucinations.

There are additional features that may be present in severe depression. Some patients exhibit a high degree of anger, for it is often suggested that depression is anger turned inwards, while paranoia is anger turned outwards. Nevertheless those who suffer from depression can be very angry with themselves, with other people and even with God for allowing them to become depressed.

There may also be an inability to concentrate; if this exhibits itself in the work situation patients have to take sick leave. If depression reveals itself in the Christian's spiritual life he may find that he cannot concentrate on Bible study or prayer, or bear to attend church.

Often, relationships deteriorate: patients become withdrawn and unable to relate to other people. This may affect their marriage, their friendships and even casual acquaintances, so that they become increasingly isolated. Some sufferers become very sensitive about the way other people behave towards them, and may become paranoid at times. Their behaviour and personality may seem to be completely altered. They may well be very retarded (slow to move or react) or on the other hand, very agitated. They feel physically ill.

Depressive neurosis

Sometimes called reactive depression, this condition has some features in common with severe depression, but sometimes differs considerably:

• The central depressive mood is more likely to become worse instead of better as the day goes on, as the day-to-day stresses increase.

• There is usually a greater element of anxiety mixed with the depression.

• The sleep disturbance is more likely to consist of initial insomnia (difficulty in falling asleep), and patients are more likely to sleep late the next day.

• Environmental precipitant – often the episode of depression has been triggered by a specific event.

• Insight is preserved – there will be no delusions or hallucinations, and patients will recognize that they are depressed, though they will still be unable to improve their condition without help.

Generally, we rightly believe that neurotic depression is a milder form of depressive illness. However, even neurotic depression can be very debilitating and cause changes in behaviour and personality. It is regarded as a "mild" condition, in so far as the whole personality is not so intensely involved, and the patient retains insight into his condition; nevertheless there will often be more anxiety present than in severe depression, and this mixture of anxiety and depression can be very distressing. Again, just as in psychotic depression, guilt will play a great part, especially for Christians.

Depression and faith

This issue of guilt is a major problem for Christians, and although I am reluctant to say so, I do feel that for this reason Christians have greater difficulty in dealing with their depression than non-Christians. Their faith is a hindrance to them rather than a help. They see the discrepancy between what they are and what they should be; between the depression they feel and the joy they should feel, and this merely aggravates their condition. Where is the joy? Where is the victory? Where is the peace beyond understanding that has been promised to us? Why do Christians find depression so hard to deal with, when they have a loving God on their side? Why does the church so often cause extra problems? All these questions require serious and prayerful consideration by the church, if it is to find ways of helping the many members of any congregation who will be struggling with this illness.

Dr David Martyn Lloyd-Jones in his book *Spiritual Depression* says, "In a sense the depressed Christian is a contradiction in terms, and is a very poor recommendation for the gospel." In saying this he shows his ignorance of the medical concept of a depressive illness. He does a great disservice to the victims who suffer from this disease, adding to their feelings of guilt and hopelessness. Depressed people need loving concern, understanding and support, not blame.

We know how common this condition is, and its victims include great and well-known personalities as well as ordinary folk. Sir Winston Churchill, that larger-than-life figure who led the country so ably through the Second World War, referred to his depression as the "black dog". St John of the Cross wrote about the "dark night of the soul". Kate Roberts, a great Welsh writer of the twentieth century, wrote a powerful novel called *Tywyll Heno* (Darkness Tonight), about the mental breakdown and recovery of a minister's wife.

William Cowper, the eighteenth-century poet who wrote some of our most treasured hymns, suffered from depression all his life. His writings reveal how a Christian with real faith in Jesus can nevertheless feel cut off from God and the church during his depressive episodes, and how, when recovering, he once again feels his connection, recognizing that his Lord shared his pain. He wrote:

> *I was a stricken deer, that left the herd*
> *Long since; with many an arrow deep infixt*
> *My panting side was charg'd, when I withdrew*
> *To seek a tranquil death in distant shades.*
> *There was I found by one who had himself*
> *Been hurt by th' archers. In his side he bore,*
> *And in his hands and feet, the cruel scars.*

Cowper's experience also enabled him to hold out the promise of hope in his hymns:

> *Ye fearful saints, fresh courage take,*
> *The clouds ye so much dread*
> *Are big with mercy, and shall break*
> *In blessings on your head.*

Yet even his faith and understanding did not protect him from recurring bouts of deep depression.

Faith is not a protection against physical disease: why should it be so against mental illness, the causes of which are still so difficult to discern? Elijah, David, Peter and Paul, heroes of our faith, all confessed that they had troubled souls and periods of depression.

When David's son Absalom committed treason and forced his ageing father to leave Jerusalem, David cried out to God: "My soul is cast down within me... all your waves and billows have gone over me... I say to God, my rock, 'Why have you forgotten me? Why must I walk about mournfully because the enemy oppresses me?'... Why are you cast down, O my soul, and why are you disquieted within me? Hope in God; for I shall again praise him, my help and my God" (Psalm 42:6, 7, 9, 11).

Peter promised faithfully that he would always remain true and faithful to his Lord, and never desert him; only a short time later he was denying Jesus, and when the cock crowed and he remembered that Jesus had predicted his betrayal, he went outside and wept bitterly.

Paul was a giant man of God, a persecutor of Christians who became a leader among them. He had seen a vision of the risen Lord that led him to bring gentiles into the kingdom by their thousands. Yet in his second letter to the church in Corinth he wrote, "We do not want you to be unaware, brothers and sisters, of the affliction we experienced in Asia; for we were so utterly, unbearably crushed that we despaired of life itself" (2 Corinthians 1:8). Later he talks of being "afflicted in every way – disputes without and fears within" (2 Corinthians 7:5).

Both Peter and Paul could be said to have suffered from reactive depression: their adverse circumstances, personal and environmental, bent them. Their personal situations – and in Peter's case, his guilt and remorse at his own actions – caused them to feel miserable, hopeless and depressed.

Elijah

Elijah was perhaps the greatest of the Old Testament prophets, and he suffered from even more severe depression, which led him to have suicidal thoughts. Like many other great men of God he experienced a moment of victory, when he must surely have felt elated: his triumph over the prophets of Baal on Mount Carmel. But after some great success, a low period often follows, and Elijah was no exception. Soon afterwards he was in despair. We can examine the elements of Elijah's depression.

Jezebel was furious that Elijah had slaughtered the prophets of Baal, and sent a message saying that she would do the same to him. Suddenly all his confidence in the Lord deserted him: "Then he was afraid; he got up and fled for his life" (1 Kings 19:3). In his anxiety and fear he surely also felt some guilt, that the vision which inspired him on Mount Carmel had deserted him. He was so depressed that only death seemed to offer respite from his pain; he felt he deserved nothing more: "It is enough; now, O Lord, take away my life, for I am no better than my ancestors" (1 Kings 19:4). He was not only fearful but suffering from an acute sense of personal failure. The effect of all this emotion was to exhaust him: he lay down under a tree and fell asleep.

We shall look later at the modern methods of treating major depressive illness. Meanwhile, we can learn a great deal by looking at the way in which God dealt with Elijah. It is noteworthy that he did not take away the source of his difficulties; nor did he resolve the problem overnight. We have to be patient when we deal with problems. I am often worried when I hear evangelists say, "Come to Jesus and all your problems will be solved." It is right that we bring all our troubles to God in prayer, but quite wrong to think that they will magically be removed. Of course it is glorious to enter into a relationship with the living Christ. When we begin to walk with him, the grass seems greener and the skies brighter: we are filled with elation. However, disillusionments and problems soon cross the new Christian's path; frustrations and fears are scattered along the way. These can multiply when the Christian lives in a non-Christian home and works in a non-Christian workplace. There may be criticism and confrontation.

When the problems come and we experience the tensions of living out our Christian life, we must not expect instant solutions. Jesus is the answer to our difficulties, but we must be patient: there may be important lessons for us to learn along the way. One is that criticisms do not only come from those outside our faith: too often Christians waste a great deal of time and energy in criticizing each other – as individuals or as denominations. As individuals and as churches we need each other's support and encouragement. We are called to work together in peace and love: "For in the one spirit we were all baptized into one body" (1 Corinthians 12:13).

This does not mean that we have to betray any central tenets of our faith, and we should certainly not compromise with the world in order to make ourselves acceptable. But we do have to have insight into each other's thoughts and feelings, and show the love of Christ towards other people, whether Christians or unbelievers. Showing love to one another is the proof of the unity of all believers, which is in turn a proof that Jesus Christ is the Son of God. What a great responsibility, and what a wonderful opportunity for healing for those who suffer emotionally, especially the depressed Christian.

When we look at the way God treated Elijah, we can observe a pattern of therapeutic steps which remain relevant today. First he allowed him to sleep, ensuring that he took proper rest. This has long been recognized as a vital tool in the treatment of depression. Before the middle of the twentieth century there were few effective therapies available, but one was narcolepsy, in which patients were given sleep-inducing drugs and allowed to sleep, sometimes for weeks. Often, when they awoke, there was a marked improvement in their condition.

Some years ago I treated a young man who had once been a member of my psychiatric team. I would have preferred another psychiatrist to see him, but he was insistent, and as he was clearly very ill I agreed to see him. I made a multiple diagnosis: he was suffering from a bleeding ulcer, hypertension and depression. His faith had all but vanished.

He was also exhausted; as we know, sleep disturbance (persistent early morning waking) is a cardinal biological symptom of major depressive illness. We began deep narcosis therapy immediately, keeping him asleep for two or three weeks altogether, though waking him for meals. We treated his physical conditions and gave him antidepressant medication, and within four months he had regained his strength and his depression had cleared. Narcosis is no longer used as a form of treatment, but it clearly had some value in this case as in the case of Elijah.

God also made sure Elijah had a proper diet: "An angel touched him and said to him, 'Get up and eat.' He looked, and there at his head was a cake baked on hot stones, and a jar of water. He ate, drank, and lay down again" (1 Kings 19:5–6). A balanced diet is vital for our mental as well as our physical health. Obesity has become a major health problem in the Western world, and there is evidence that hyperactivity and lack of concentration in children can be traced to a poor diet. Thousands of years ago God showed Elijah that he needed to look after his basic well-being by eating regular meals.

Next, God gave him hope. "Get up and eat, otherwise the journey will be too much for you" (1 Kings 19:7). He was to go on a journey for God: there was still purpose in his life, and God had work for him to do. He must have felt valued by God, and this is another important gift that we can give those who suffer in this way.

When Elijah had travelled for forty days and nights he arrived at Mount Horeb, or Sinai, where Moses received the Ten Commandments from God. Simply by being in this special and holy place he was reminded of the history of his people and the faithfulness of God. Then God spoke to Elijah directly – not in the wind, not in the earthquake, not in the fire, but in the silence that followed. He caused him to re-evaluate his ministry: "'What are you doing here, Elijah?'… 'I have been very zealous for the Lord'" (1 Kings 19:13–14). He realized that he had indeed been faithful, and that his ministry was worthwhile.

Lessons from God

This story offers comfort to the Christian who suffers from depression. It shows that however far we may feel from God, he will return and speak to us again, and grant us even more blessings and an even greater ministry. Elijah was promised a glorious task: to anoint Jehu, the future king of Israel, and Elisha, his own successor. He was given an undertaking that God would be victorious and all his enemies would be destroyed. He might have felt lost and alone ("I alone am left, and they are seeking my life") but when he was restored to health, God was able to point out to him that he had never been alone; there were 7,000 others in Israel who had never lost their faith and had never bowed down to Baal.

When people become depressed, isolation can be one of their greatest problems – they hesitate to inflict their low moods on other people, and their friends may avoid them because they cannot find anything to say that will help. I knew a young mother of three who was suffering from post-natal depression. She remarked that while she was in the maternity ward she had lots of visitors, sharing in her happiness and bringing her good wishes. Once she was admitted to a psychiatric ward there were no visits – people were embarrassed or afraid to come and see her. Her minister, when asked, gave the excuse that he "didn't want to interfere with her treatment". She told me that while she was in hospital all she wanted was for the minister or a member of her church to come and visit her, to show her that she was still loved and accepted, and to remind her that neither they nor God had forgotten her.

As Christians we should recognize the importance of visiting the sufferers, sharing our faith, praying with and for them, and showing our love and concern. This helps to reassure them that God still loves and cares for them, and that this is demonstrated through the church; that they are not alone, but that there are thousands of others who keep the faith with them.

Elijah, David, Peter and Paul were no less men of God because they suffered from depression. The suggestion in *Spiritual Depression* that such people are a poor advertisement for the gospel is as foolish as suggesting that we let God down if we catch a cold. If I can convince one depressed Christian that this is so, this book will achieve something. Even when Christians feel they have lost their faith, God continues to have an interest in them, loves them and wants to sustain them. Elijah had been suicidally depressed, but now he was given new goals to rebuild the nation. Modern sufferers can be assured that God will restore their faith and cause them to rise again, that they will have a purpose in life and continue to serve him. Pastors and church members should consider it their duty and joy to stand beside their suffering brothers and sisters, to hold them up and provide them with the strength to keep the hope of recovery alive.

Notes

1 A. Hale, "ABC of mental health: depression", *British Medical Journal*, 315 (5 July 1997), pp. 43-46, quoted in MIND factsheet.

2 L. Bird, *The Fundamental Facts* (London: Mental Health Foundation, 1999), quoted in MIND factsheet.

3 Source: The Mental Health Foundation.

4 Source: The Mental Health Foundation.

5 G.E. Murphy, "Social origins of depression in old age", British Journal of Psychiatry, 141, (1982), pp. 135-42.

6 A.F. Jorn, "The epidemiology of depressive states in the elderly", *Social Psychiatry and Psychiatric Epidemiology*, 30 (1995), pp. 53-59.

7 F. Goodwin & K. Jamison, *Manic-depressive Illness* (Oxford: OUP, 1990), quoted in MIND factsheet.

8 Source: The Mental Health Foundation.

9 Source: The Mental Health Foundation.

10 National Patient Safety Agency, *Safety First, National Confidential Inquiry into Suicide and Homicide by People with Mental Illness* (2001), quoted in MIND factsheet.

11 Source: Office for National Statistics.

5

CHURCH OR CLINIC?

Over the last fifty years or so there has been a revolution in the treatment of psychiatric disorders. Before the 1950s there was little or no effective treatment: anxious or manic patients could be sedated; depressed patients could be given stimulants such as amphetamines. However, around this time there were great advances in drug therapy, with the development of antidepressants and antipsychotic medication; this was accompanied by great strides forward in the area of psychotherapy.

One might have expected that sufferers would welcome these advances, but there have always been difficulties in the treatment of those with mental illness. First there is the reluctance to accept the diagnosis, mainly because of the stigma that attaches to mental illness, which was discussed earlier. This reluctance may also be manifested in an unwillingness to be referred to a psychiatrist. Even when this is achieved, and the psychiatrist has succeeded in outlining a course of treatment, there is usually a problem with compliance. Patients may be unwilling to undertake their treatment – whether it is medication or psychotherapy – and once persuaded to do so, may fail to complete the course.

Healing

Christians, in particular, often fail in this respect. They say that they would rather rely on God for their healing, and turn to their minister and their church fellowship for prayer, rejecting medical help. Although such people usually have no difficulty in accepting that they would have to use insulin to control diabetes, should they develop it, they remain reluctant to accept the standard treatment for their depression or anxiety. It is almost as if they have fallen prey to the old myths we were looking at earlier: that mental illness is in some sense less "real" than other physical illnesses, and that recovery can be more easily achieved by other means.

People have often asked me, "Can't people who suffer mental illness be healed through prayer and laying-on of hands, just as others are?" The answer is "Certainly they can." Nothing is beyond our God. "Is any one of you sick? He should call the elders of the church to pray over him and anoint him with oil in the name of the Lord. And the prayer offered in faith will make the sick person well; the Lord will raise him up" (James 5:14–15). We all know of wonderful miracles of healing, and we praise God for them. Yet we must be honest and admit that we also know of cases when people have not been healed, and we do not know the reason why. Kathryn Kuhlman, who had a healing ministry, once replied to a journalist who asked her why some people were not healed. She said that she didn't know. One day, when she got to heaven, she would ask Jesus, but meanwhile she went on faithfully doing his will, and laying on hands and praying for the sick.

Tragically, some healers become convinced that everyone can be healed if only they have enough faith. When someone comes for prayer and is not healed, they may suggest that it is the patient's own fault: he has insufficient faith. This is a cruel thing to say to anyone, especially someone who is already suffering.

Healing is a complex and difficult subject, but we must

not shirk the task of thinking about it prayerfully. We know that God can and does heal people – but he uses a variety of means. He may heal in answer to prayer. He has also given us the tools for healing many of our own ills. He has given us minds to think with, and hands to work with, and we accept his gifts with joy and thankfulness. We thank him for the talents and skills of musicians who help us to praise him; for the abilities of scientists and inventors who have discovered the many wonders of our world, making life better for millions of people. Why should we stop at the abilities of doctors? The expertise and knowledge of the psychiatrist, the drugs that have been discovered and the therapeutic techniques that have been developed, are just as much the gifts of God, made available to us through his creation, to help us to alleviate suffering.

The Christian psychiatrist

Once patients have accepted the need for treatment and the referral, they enter into a therapeutic relationship with the psychiatrist. They must feel able to share their doubts and fears with the practitioner, about the form of treatment, its possible side effects, and how far it can be reconciled with their Christian faith. At this point we reach the fundamental question that was posed at the beginning of this book: is it acceptable for Christians to say that they want to be treated only by a Christian psychiatrist? Can a Christian be treated appropriately by a non-Christian?

As a psychiatrist and a Christian I have a heart for people and I care about their feelings. I appreciate that my Christian patients have very specific fears that often narrow their understanding. They may have struggled to accept their illness and they may have just about managed to resign themselves to the need for treatment, but they then demand to see a Christian psychiatrist. There are usually two motivations – one is reasonable, and the other less so. Firstly, they feel that a Christian psychiatrist will respect their faith and not mock them or suggest that it is an irrational belief. Secondly, they may feel that as a Christian brother or sister, the psychiatrist will be more susceptible to pressure from the patient not to do anything they dislike – delivering unwelcome diagnoses or dispensing drugs. This is the less reasonable aspect: a good psychiatrist will not allow his or her professional conduct to be dictated by the prejudices of the patient.

The answer to this is quite clear. What patients need is a physician in psychological medicine who is competent, understanding and able to gather facts, make an accurate diagnosis and then set out a management and treatment plan. The doctor will bring into this all the relevant modern treatments, whether drugs or psychotherapy, and take into account all the social and religious aspects of the patient's life. It would be absolutely no use to have a doctor who was a good Christian but a poor psychiatrist. As a Christian I believe that God wants me to be good at my job, to do my duty and to act professionally at all times. My colleagues (whether they believe in God or not) operate on the same professional principles. My Christian faith inevitably affects how I manage and treat people, and of course I am able to empathize with the particular concerns of Christian patients. But there is no reason to suppose that a competent non-Christian psychiatrist would not be able to manage a Christian patient.

In every case, the faith aspects will be considered and their relevance assessed. If patients feel that their faith is not being taken into account then they have the right to express their dissatisfaction. The psychiatrist can then assure them that he is competent to deal with this, that he accepts that their faith is real to them and that he will attempt to mobilize it in a positive way in the course of the treatment. If there is any doubt in the psychiatrist's mind that he is able to deal comfortably with the matter of the patient's faith, then the appropriate procedure would be for him to refer the patient to another psychiatrist who would be able to handle this aspect better.

It must be underlined that it is never acceptable for a psychiatrist to abuse someone's faith or make fun of it or fail to take it seriously. The only time I have ever interfered with a colleague's handling of a case was when I knew that they dealt with a patient in this manner – it is quite indefensible. All psychiatrists are trained to take into account social, cultural and religious issues – indeed, one of the most recent textbooks on the subject is called *A Handbook of Psychiatry – a South Asian perspective*,[1] and it deals with the specific issues arising from that particular culture.

Specific fears

Having said this, it may be true that a psychiatrist who is a committed Christian may have more to offer a Christian patient. Christians often have specific fears concerning their treatment. They often have more resistance to drug therapies than other patients, because they believe (wrongly) that all antidepressants are addictive; they generally have the idea that "drugs are bad for you"; and especially because they cling to the myth that accepting any form of treatment is a sign of weakness or lack of faith.

In fact compliance is an issue to a certain extent with all patients. Some research has shown that around 50 per cent of patients do not take their drugs as prescribed. There is a danger of patients being prescribed antidepressants for months on end because their condition has not improved;

in fact they may be taking the drugs haphazardly or not at all, and if they followed the prescription the treatment could be successfully completed much sooner.

There is also a tendency for people to take their antidepressants, find that their condition improves, and then discontinue the medication suddenly, resulting in a rapid relapse of their depressive symptomology. This can be avoided if a doctor or nurse takes the time to give patients a full explanation, answering questions and assuaging their fears.

Christians also tend to have enhanced suspicions of psychotherapies, or "talking cures". They fear that they will be "brainwashed" or hypnotized, that their free will may be taken away from them, and that they will be imbued with secular thinking and their faith diluted. Once again, these fears can be assuaged by proper information and a health professional who takes the time to answer questions with patience and understanding. If patients respect and trust the psychiatrist they are much more likely to comply with their treatment and it has a much greater chance of success.

Spiritual awareness

The Christian is not alone in saying, in effect, "I want to be understood by my doctor." Everyone has the right to be treated by a competent professional who has the entire armament available – including the ability to recognize his or her own prejudices, if any.

However, there is one area in which the Christian psychiatrist has an extra ability at his fingertips: he has the potential for spiritual awareness, and the ability to offer (if it is requested) spiritual direction. The non-Christian psychiatrist cannot do this: he or she does not accept the possibility and has no access to the great truths of the faith as found in scripture and the history of the faithful. The Christian psychiatrist may be asked by a Christian patient if they might pray together, and I always agree to this, though I would never initiate it.

Indeed, I have had some Christian patients who fail to understand either my profession or my faith, who have said, "Just pray for me and I'll pay you your fee – then there'll be no need for me to go through therapy." This always reminds me of the story of Simon the Sorcerer: "Now when Simon saw that the Spirit was given through the laying on of the apostles' hands, he offered them money, saying, 'Give me also this power so that anyone on whom I lay my hands may receive the Holy Spirit'" (Acts 8:18–9). The secret of faith is not for sale, and certainly the process of psychiatric treatment cannot be bypassed in such a way.

One does occasionally come across cases where depression or somatoform conditions are resistant to either drug treatment or psychotherapy, but where in the course of discussion between patient and doctor a different problem is revealed. I once treated a woman for persistent facial pain for which no physical cause was found. One day during her psychotherapy she burst into tears and admitted that she had not seen her only son for ten years, and had never seen his children. She had quarrelled with him over his wedding and neither she nor her husband had attended it. No amount of psychotherapy would have improved her condition until this underlying issue was attended to. A Christian can readily understand this, and see the remedy in terms of the process of forgiveness and the removal of guilt. She needed spiritual direction and advice to be reconciled with her son before she could find peace within herself and before God.

Other patients have asked me to pray with them for forgiveness and relief from guilt; when we have done this, and it is clear that they have repented before God, their guilt and their psychological symptoms leave them symultaneously. Often my consulting room has become a "house of prayer". I have seen patients forget my presence as a therapist as they make peace with God. Jesus promised that where two or three are gathered in his name, he will be there among them. He does come to bless and heal.

Common ground

Most people who suffer from emotional difficulties want to learn about their condition. It is very important that they have access to the doctors and others involved in their treatment, to discuss their illness and all the other issues surrounding it. There are also excellent resources available on the internet, especially from MIND, the mental health organisation, and others, which also produce information leaflets and other printed materials (see the section on Useful Addresses at the back of this book). Conferences, public meetings, question-and-answer sessions, consumer groups and patient advocacy groups all provide important support; they help to break down barriers and erase the stigma.

The church is also a place where this kind of work should go on, where people can get involved with helping sufferers and where information can be disseminated. Support for those suffering from mental illness is a bridge that church members can cross to meet those in need in the world outside. So often sufferers can feel isolated and alone: where better to go than a church, whose members are committed to following their Lord in reaching out to the lost and lonely? In cases of chronic mental illness there is a need for long-term support: where better to find it than a church, whose members are prepared to serve with great patience and persistence?

Christians (whether sufferers or carers) should never feel that there is any conflict between the Christian faith and the principles of clinical psychiatry – if there were, I should not have been able to conduct my professional life and obey my calling as a Christian for so many years. In fact there is a great deal of common ground between the two, enabling me to speak the same language with confidence with both my colleagues and my Christian patients.

Respect for mankind

Physicians and Christians share the belief that every individual is of great worth, no matter how he behaves. The physician may deplore the fact that the patient does things which damage his health (smoking, drinking or indulging in risky behaviour); the Christian may deplore the facts of sin and failure; yet both persevere in his care, whether to heal or to save. Doctors and nurses will labour to save the life and improve the health of everyone – the very old, the drug addict, and the terminally ill patient. Everyone is of worth. The Christian sees in everyone a reflection of God's Spirit, made in his image, and valuable in his sight. For this person Jesus surrendered himself voluntarily on the cross, so that his sins might be set aside and he could be reconciled to God. How can we not care for this person, so precious to God?

Wholeness

The psychiatrist is in a sense the complete physician, in that he takes the whole person into consideration, both physical and psychological. Psychiatry emphasizes the interaction of body and mind, the importance of psychological factors in the production of physical disease, and the physical causes of psychological illness. The Christian finds this an easy concept to accept: running through the New Testament is a common strand that emphasizes the unity of body, mind and spirit, and the need to restore wholeness. Paul in his epistles stresses the need to be strong in body, sane in mind and mature in spirit. Wholeness means healing, and psychiatry concurs. (We consider this topic in more detail in Chapter 10.)

Relationships

Both Christianity and psychiatry focus on the supreme importance of relationships. Psychotherapy is unique among medical procedures in its wide-ranging treatment of the whole person rather than a specific attack on the symptoms of a disease alone. It takes into account the patient's family, friends and entire social world. It insists that relationships are important to a person's health, and the Christian agrees. Whether we think of the story of the Good Samaritan ("Who is my neighbour?") or the advice of the writers of the epistles, over and over again we see that relationships with other people are vital to the spiritual well-being of the individual and the church. Ultimately, of course, the Christian believes in one relationship that is greater than all others: our relationship with God.

Flawed minds

In psychiatry we are trying to change sick minds; they need changing because they are flawed. Every human being has the potential for both good and bad, and the New Testament sums this up from a different angle: "All have sinned and fall short of the glory of God" (Romans 3:23). Any system of psychiatry that attempts to operate without taking into account the commonly accepted obligations in a moral society will be incomplete.

Guilt

Both psychiatry and Christianity recognize and try to deal with most people's greatest burden: guilt. Psychiatry differentiates pathological guilt (which may be a symptom of a depressive illness and will disappear when the illness is cured) from normal guilt (a reaction to some past misdemeanour). Christians recognize that theological guilt (where a person feels that he has sinned against God and deserves punishment) may be based on fact, and nothing will clear it but the acceptance of Christ's atoning death.

Sexual health

Psychiatry has sometimes been wrongly blamed for advocating sexual freedom and encouraging promiscuity. In fact, psychiatry advocates a healthy attitude towards sex and more open discussion about it, but it never suggests that promiscuity will lead to health and happiness. Rather, it teaches that order, discipline and respect for others is the basis for healthy and successful living. In the same way, people have criticized the church for being rigid, reactionary and hypocritical about sex, when in fact Christians believe that sex is a gift from God. At the heart of the marital relationship it brings great joy.

Love

Finally, both Christianity and psychiatry share a belief in the importance of love. Love and empathy are at the heart of the advances in my own profession; they are crucial in our relationships with patients. A loving concern is an essential ingredient in all our dealing with those who suffer. Every patient needs the loving support of other people; without it, the road to recovery is long and lonely and very hard. Christians share this belief: Christ's great commandment was that we should love one another. It is Christ's love that inspires our Christian living and our relationships with other people.

The importance of diagnosis

We have seen that Christians need not fear psychiatry, whether or not their practitioner is also a Christian. The central tenets of the faith are not denied by the assumptions of psychiatry, and no doctor would ask a patient to do or believe anything that was contrary to the essentials of their faith. It is vital that such fears do not prevent Christians from seeking the treatment they need.

By the time anyone meets a psychiatrist for the first time, they will probably have already realized that they are suffering from a mental illness of some sort. They may have approached their GP in the first instance (the most common source of referrals); or they may have seen a member of the community mental health team such as the community psychiatric nurse. Occasionally they may have taken the first step by visiting a counselling service such as Cruse (the bereavement service), Relate (who deal with relationship difficulties) or even the Citizens Advice Bureau (who help with all kinds of problems, including financial ones). All these agencies have staff who are trained to spot the symptoms that suggest that a medical consultation might be helpful, and they will usually suggest a visit to the GP for the preliminary diagnosis.

Once a person has been referred to a psychiatrist, the first and most important step is the initial assessment. Sometimes it may be necessary to interview the patient on more than one occasion for a definite diagnosis to be made. First a history will be taken, including the patient's personal development, education, psychosexual history, medical and psychiatric history, religious history, forensic history if applicable, and the history of the present illness, with its onset, any associated stresses and obvious causes, and the development of the symptomology.

The second part of the initial assessment will be an examination of the mental state and, if appropriate, the physical state. The mental state examination will cover such elements as behaviour, mood or emotions, and also the content of the thoughts, especially if there are any delusions or hallucinations. Cognitive functions will be checked, including orientation, attention, concentration and memory. The doctor will note how good the patient's insight is, the intelligence and what kind of rapport has been established.

If a physical examination seems necessary, the relevant blood tests etc. will be done, along with weight and height measurements. The patient will be asked about alcohol consumption, appetite and any changes in sleep patterns. There will be questions about any drugs taken (whether prescribed, over-the-counter, or illegal). Increasingly these days patients may have tried a range of alternative treatments, ranging from herbal remedies to acupuncture, in an attempt to improve their health. These must be identified; patients sometimes think herbal medicines are not relevant because they are marketed as "natural" remedies, but they can have very powerful effects, and may interact with any other medication that is prescribed.

This interview will take up to an hour and a half, and at

the end the patient and the psychiatrist together will discuss the possible diagnosis.

It cannot be emphasized enough that diagnosis is the first step to the proper management and treatment of mental illness. Some critics have expressed doubt about the possibility of a firm diagnosis in mental illness, and queried the validity of the classification systems we use. There is continual discussion about these labels for mental states, but the system is the best we have. It may not be perfect; often the boundaries between classifications are somewhat blurred; many patients present with a mixture of symptoms (such as anxiety combined with depression); yet it produces workable categorizations and enables us to treat people with great success.

Often the diagnosis alone is an effective tool in producing an improvement in the way people feel. Time and time again I have explained to patients that they are suffering from a depressive illness, and that this is a physiological and psychological condition: the description cannot fully explain the hell they feel they are going through, but there are treatments available. They are immensely reassured by this: often even the depressive tries to smile for the first time in months.

I have also seen the tragedies that occur when people have entered into psychotherapy or group therapy without adequate assessment and before a diagnosis has been made. Patients who are referred for group therapy for schizophrenic symptoms will not improve and will probably worsen. If they had been properly assessed in the first place by a psychiatrist and diagnosed with acute schizophrenia, they would have been treated with the appropriate antipsychotic medication which generally brings about an improvement in a very short time.

Psychiatrists and churches both need to take care when

patients or church members describe their "spiritual" symptoms. The tendency is to assume that the patient requires a diagnosis that embraces the specifically spiritual aspects, but in fact the religious element may well be delusional; the illness may be simply diagnosed as depression or other psychotic condition, and the spiritual problems disappear as the illness improves under treatment. One man of my acquaintance complained of his inability to read scripture or to pray, but it was clear that he was suffering from a severe depressive illness. After medication and psychotherapy he recovered from his depression, and his spiritual life was restored at the same time. He was relieved when he came to realize that his illness was a mental disorder with a spiritual aspect to it, and when he had a recurrence he would come to the hospital and seek treatment himself.

Churches often find themselves in a great deal of confusion when Christians suggest that they are possessed. One young man came to me in this condition, saying that his church had conducted a session of exorcism for him, subjecting him to hours of prayer. Not only had this not helped him, but he felt much worse and markedly more guilty: surely he must be beyond help if this spiritual procedure had failed to cast out his demons? He was diagnosed as suffering from a depressive illness with accompanying delusions; he received antidepressant medication and supportive psychotherapy and recovered completely. He has remained well for several years.

I am not saying that there is no place for the church: it is right to ask for healing and to support sufferers with prayer. But a great deal of damage can be done if there has not been a proper medical diagnosis: imagine the results if churches routinely insisted on prayer for stomach-ache when the person was suffering from appendicitis.

Christians often suffer from increased guilt when they discuss their condition with church leaders, because they are made to feel that their psychological symptoms are a sign of weakness or of sin. Some famous Christians have misguidedly suggested that sin is a cause of depression, and thereby caused great suffering.

Some patients bring their relationship difficulties into the fellowship and consequently cause trouble in their church. Symptoms associated with depression are irritability and increased sensitivity – at times verging on paranoia – and this can often cause rifts with other church members. These people may in any case have fundamental personality traits that have been present for most of their lives, that make it difficult for them to make or sustain relationships. I once knew a neurological registrar with a great deal of insight: she had developed manic depression, but she said that she had always been miserable and depressed as a result of difficulties in her childhood and the disruption of her family life. She could see that her manic depressive psychosis was grafted on to a chronically miserable personality.

Obsessive personalities, as we observed earlier, are made more vulnerable to depressive illness by their perfectionism and insistence on having everything "right". John Bunyan and Martin Luther are examples of Christian perfectionists who suffered in this way. Churches should always be aware that when prayer and scripture reading become difficult, or a Christian finds it impossible to take part in worship and fellowship, this may well be the distressing result of a depressive illness, and this possibility should be explored by a doctor.

A woman once came to my surgery and said, "I've come for a happiness pill." There is no such thing. There is no medication that will remove all the stresses and strains of life, and God forbid that there should ever be such a thing. Should all unhappiness be regarded as an illness to be cured? I do not believe so. Christians know that they are not immune to the troubles of everyday life, and that God may be teaching them valuable lessons through them. Nevertheless, depression and other mental disorders are illnesses, and doctors have the privilege and the responsibility of diagnosing these conditions, and working to alleviate suffering wherever we can.

Notes

1 Dinesh Bhugra, Gopinath Ranjith and Vikram Patel, *A Handbook of Psychiatry – a South Asian Perspective* (Tunbridge Wells: Anshan Ltd, 2005).

6

GETTING HELP

If you think you or a member of your family may be suffering from mental illness, where can you get help? It is useful to know something about the practitioners who will be helping you, and the places where you may receive treatment.

The practitioners

Patients may come into contact with many different people who are involved in their care, because the National Health Service has developed systems for delivering the full range of mental health services on a local basis. All Primary Care Trusts must appoint staff and put mechanisms in place to ensure that patients suffering from mental illnesses are recognized and referred promptly for specialist help.[1]

GPs

The general practitioner should always be the first port of call. They usually know the medical and family background, which gives them a great advantage in assessing the patient's condition. They will discuss their problems in the setting of their personal and family life. All GPs have some training in mental health care, and they are able to consider the best form of management and treatment: they can prescribe appropriate medication and/or give helpful advice for the more common conditions. They are also the gatekeepers for specialist services: their preliminary diagnosis will indicate whether a referral is necessary, and suggest which is the appropriate consultant or other specialist for this.

In Britain 98 per cent of people are registered with a GP. Around 70 per cent of registered patients will consult their doctor in a given year, and up to 20 per cent of the GP's time is taken up with mental health and related problems. Most people are generally satisfied with the service they receive: around 90 per cent think their GP communicates well with them, and 80 per cent think their GP generally makes the right diagnosis.[2] Once a person has contacted a GP, their needs are usually met within the practice: fewer than 10 per cent of cases require referral to specialist care within the mental health services.

However, it is important to note that an estimated one in four people suffering from a mental illness have not consulted a professional about that illness. This may be partly due to the stigma attached to it, and is another reason why seeing the GP is a good first step. There is no stigma attached to visiting the local surgery, and there is a very good chance that treatment will be completed in that environment.

Community mental health teams

Community mental health teams are designed to provide a full range of support for people suffering from mental illness, and also for their carers. The team may include health professionals such as psychiatrists and psychologists, mental health nurses, occupational therapists and counsellors provided by the NHS, and also social workers and other carers provided by the local authority.

Psychiatric nurses may work in psychiatric hospitals or day hospitals, but some also work in the community, when they are known as community mental health nurses. They are registered mental nurses who have their own training, and they can provide long-term support, see patients regularly to talk about their condition and suggest coping methods, and give some medication.

Counselling may be provided by specialist counsellors; however, it can also be delivered by other professionals such as social workers, mental health nurses, psychotherapists and occupational therapists.

Social workers provide practical advice on issues such as finance, applying for benefits and finding accommodation. Approved social workers are specially trained and may be authorized under the Mental Health Act (1983) to recommend a compulsory stay in hospital if they think someone is at risk.

If there are several people involved in helping the patient, it is likely that a care co-ordinator (or keyworker) will be assigned. This helps to ensure that there is a single point of contact; they liaise with the rest of the team and make sure that both patient and carers know what everyone is doing. They work alongside the patient to draw up a care plan and make sure that everyone has a copy, so that patients know what support they will get.

Psychiatrists

There is a surprising amount of confusion about the different roles in specialist mental health care, partly because the names sound similar to those outside the profession, and partly because some of the titles are applied to both medical and lay practitioners. Psychiatrists are physicians who have qualified in medicine and then proceeded to advanced training in the diagnosis and treatment of mental and emotional disorders. This leads to a higher qualification and in particular to membership of the Royal College of Psychiatrists. Like all doctors, they have completed all their preliminary training before entering the senior house officer grade for training in psychological medicine. They then become specialist registrars in psychiatry.

Their studies involve general adult psychiatry, child psychiatry, social and rehabilitative psychiatry, psychotherapy and forensic psychiatry; they gain knowledge of the law as it relates to mental health, and generally go on to specialize in one particular discipline, such as psychogeriatric medicine (dealing with mental illness in the elderly).

Psychotherapists

All psychiatrists practise some psychotherapy, but some specialize in this field and become psychotherapists. Psychotherapy is a form of "talking cure": the patient talks to the doctor, who intervenes and contributes when necessary. Psychotherapy is communication in a specially supportive setting: it is important that there is trust and empathy in the relationship between doctor and patient. It may be done in one-to-one situations or groups; it may be superficial (as in counselling), supportive (allowing the patient to share problems and worries and helping them to feel that they are understood in a supportive relationship), or deep (aiming to effect change in the person). Research indicates that the personality of the psychotherapist is important in achieving successful outcomes: warmth, understanding and confidentiality are essential.

There are also lay psychotherapists who are not psychiatrists, and have no medical training. Some have recognized qualifications and are members of one of the recognized bodies (such as the British Association of Counsellors and Psychotherapists or the UK Council for Psychotherapy).

Psychoanalysts

Psychoanalysis is a particular form of psychotherapy; it follows the theory of Sigmund Freud, which divides the mental life into conscious and unconscious, and uses a special technique of free association, in which patients are encouraged to talk about anything that comes to mind, expressing their feelings and ideas at will. From this unguarded conversation the therapists can often discover conflicts that are hidden deep in the unconscious mind, of which the patient may be unaware. Past feelings and attitudes may be brought to light and thus transferred from the unconscious to the conscious mind, where they can be discussed, dealt with and changed. Once again, all psychoanalysts have first studied psychotherapy, but not all psychotherapists practice psychoanalysis. Jung's form of psychoanalysis embraces the spritual element as indicated later in Chapter 8.

Psychologists

Clinical psychologists have studied the academic discipline of psychology, traditionally defined as the "science of mind", but increasingly in recent years as the "science of behaviour". They usually have a degree in psychology and then undertake further training in the diagnosis and treatment of mental illness. They are primarily concerned with the ways in which people think, act and manage their relationships. They may use psychotherapy and other specialized assessment techniques, usually working under medical supervision.

Psychiatrists and psychologists are all professionally trained. However, psychiatrists are medically trained, and as doctors are able to prescribe medication. Psychologists are not medically trained, and do not use drugs in treatment. Only a psychiatrist can physically examine a patient and thus deal with the whole person, including both physical and mental symptoms. Only a psychiatrist can become a Responsible Medical Officer under the terms of the Mental Health Act (1983).

Treatment centres

Many types of services are available to people who experience mental health problems, and they may be referred from a variety of starting points: not just the GP but hospital accident and emergency departments, the police, the probation service, the prison service, and services for the homeless.

Hospitals

Hospitals provide a range of services, from outpatient clinics through day hospitals to inpatient care in psychiatric wards in general hospitals. There are still some specialist hospitals providing psychiatric care, but nowadays these are becoming rarer: many of the old institutions (often set up in the nineteenth century) are being closed down.

The old distinction between psychiatric and general hospitals was removed by the 1959 Mental Health Act, when the treatment of patients in the community was first suggested. It became easier to treat patients at home when the new psychotropic drugs were developed in the 1960s. The number of NHS beds for mental illness began to reduce sharply in the 1970s, and it has continued to fall steadily. In Wales, the number of beds in the mental health sector fell by 43 per cent over the ten years from 1994 to 2004.[3] In Scotland, the number of beds fell from 13,796 in 1990 to 7,561 in 2000.[4] In England, the average daily number of beds in NHS facilities fell by 10 per cent (almost 4,000 beds) over the five years to 2000.[5]

The emphasis has shifted from caring for patients in hospitals to keeping them in their own homes and treating them in the community. Nevertheless, hospitalization still accounts for about 75 per cent of NHS spending on mental health.[6] There are always some people who need either care for acute conditions (they are generally admitted to hospital in a crisis for a short stay), or longer-term treatment and care (they may spend longer in hospital or have several short stays over a long period). Hospitals can be a place of refuge for some seriously ill patients who find coping in the world "outside" too much for them. They also provide opportunities for staff to assess their needs and try to find the best ways of helping them.

At times admission to hospital is the treatment of choice, because the patient is thus taken out of a stressful (often family) situation, to the relief of all concerned. This allows both patient and family a "cooling-off" period, thus avoiding an escalation of stress and possibly even violence.

There is occasionally criticism of the "revolving door" situation, where patients come in and out of hospital, but this is not necessarily a bad thing. If it is a definite policy decision that a patient needs repeated short stays over a period, then the situation is controlled. The problems arise only with those patients who are discharged – or insist on discharging themselves – before their condition has improved, and who then relapse and have to be readmitted: in that case the situation is uncontrolled and clearly benefits neither the patient nor the hospital's management of the case.

Certainly the figures show a trend for shorter stays in hospital. The mean duration of stay for the mentally ill was nearly 55 days in 2001–2002, half the number it was in 1991–1992. Stays for acute patients are generally much shorter: in 2000–2001, acute patients stayed in hospital for an average of 5.1 days, though in 1991–1992 it was 6 days.[7]

Most people go into hospital on an informal basis, but there are a number (around 15 per cent) of compulsory admissions, where people are detained under the Mental Health Act (1983). Strict criteria must be met before anyone can be detained in this way. There are various scenarios: patients may be admitted for assessment or treatment or both; the application may be made by a relative or the authorized social worker, or occasionally by a court. In all cases two doctors must confirm that the patient is suffering from a relevant mental disorder and that he or she ought to be detained in the interests of his or her own health or safety, or in order to protect others. (In cases of emergency, one doctor's signature will suffice.) Strict time limits are laid down for the period of detention.

To "section" a patient (i.e. to detain them under the relevant section of the Mental Health Act) can be a most effective therapeutic measure at a critical phase in the course of an illness. It should certainly never be regarded as punishment.

Residential care

There are other alternatives for patients who feel unable to manage their lives unaided. For long-term requirements, residential care homes offer a safe and supportive environment for people with severe mental health problems. People with milder conditions may choose to live independently in rented accommodation in supported housing schemes, where they have the help of a mental health support worker. For short-term needs there are hostels that offer accommodation with some supervision, and there are also some therapeutic communities that provide a rehabilitation programme and group or individual therapy for residents.

Community services

The closure of the traditional psychiatric hospitals has inevitably led to a change in the way that mental health services are provided. Community mental health teams (as described above) are an example of this. A wider range of services is provided by a number of different agencies and professionals, drawn from both the health service and the local authority. These may include social clubs, support services (including targeted support for particular conditions or minority ethnic groups), advocacy services, and help with housing and employment. Day centres provide recreation as well as the opportunity for social interaction and some therapy.

The development of such services has greatly improved the experience of patients with mental illness, allowing them to receive the proper treatment alongside rehabilitative activities, reducing the threat of social isolation. However, there have also been significant gaps in the service. There are indications that, for some patients (such as those suffering from schizophrenia), the contact they had with the community psychiatric nurse provided inadequate support: sometimes this consisted of a fortnightly injection. As a result, approximately half the patients with schizophrenia lost contact with specialist mental health services, with consequences ranging from severe relapses into illness to homelessness.

In a bid to change this situation, a new development in community provision is "assertive outreach", where teams focus on the needs of people with severe mental illness. Evidence suggests that an assertive outreach team can provide a more effective service to people who are reluctant to engage with mental health services and who require long-term intensive support. The provision may include day-to-day engagement and active help care or rehabilitation. An economic analysis has revealed that providing such support is more cost-effective than uncontrolled "revolving door" hospital admissions or twenty-four-hour nursing care.

Counselling services

Counselling is a superficial form of psychotherapy, and it can be extremely effective. It is so useful that over 50 per cent of GP surgeries have qualified and approved counsellors attached to their practice.[8]

There are also counsellors who set up private practices, which people may choose to attend without a referral. Some are very good at what they do, but it is important to know that it is possible to set up a business as a "counsellor" with no qualifications at all. There are many such people operating in this way, with varying degrees of success and effectiveness. Indeed many ordinary people, who have no training even in counselling, successfully perform a similar service for their family and friends in an informal way, by listening to their problems and difficulties and allowing them to talk and find their way to solutions. A similar activity occurs in self-help groups such as Alcoholics Anonymous.

This is an area where the church can be of great help. There is a grey area between "counselling" and "befriending", and the church is ideally placed to offer support across the whole spectrum of need. There is now an Association of Christian Counsellors to which both Christians and non-Christians can be referred, and it is helpful for churches to know that this kind of support is available. We explore the implications in Chapter 9 of this book.

Notes

1 The National Service Framework for Mental Health, 1999.
2 The National Survey of NHS Patients in General Practice, 1998.
3 National Assembly for Wales, *Statistical Release 61/2004: NHS Beds 2003-4*.
4 Information Services Department, NHS National Services Scotland.
5 Department of Health.
6 Dr Andrew Thompson, "Patterns of admission for adult psychiatric illness in England: analysis of Hospital Episode Statistics Data", *British Journal of Psychiatry*, 185 (2004), pp 334-341.
7 Office for National Statistics.
8 Mental After Care Association, *First National GP Survey of Mental Health Aftercare* (1999). Available at www.together-uk.org/index

7

TREATMENTS

Mental illness has always been recognized as a disorder afflicting large numbers of individuals in society. Sadly, in the past it was imperfectly understood and carried the stigma of danger and fear that accompanied the brutal label of "insanity". Those few who were very ill were incarcerated in the gloomy institutions known as "insane asylums"; lesser conditions such as anxiety or depression were scarcely recognized as illnesses, and sufferers were left to cope as best they could – and often greeted with the purposeless phrase, "Pull yourself together."

It was only in the early years of the twentieth century that Freud began to develop his insight that there was a division between the conscious and unconscious mind, which could affect feelings and behaviour. He developed methods of psychoanalysis in which people were encouraged to talk about their thoughts and feelings, and in the process uncover memories or ideas which they had repressed. This activity helped many people to deal with their problems and overcome anxiety, depression and other conditions. Over the years his ideas were built upon (and sometimes argued over) by other people, who developed different schools of psychoanalysis and psychotherapy.

Meanwhile other scientific advances in the understanding of brain chemistry brought about a change in attitudes to mental illness. The concept of neurobiological origins for psychiatric disorders had two effects: it began to destigmatize mental illnesses (once they could be seen as diseases like any other) and it encouraged the search for pharmaceutical remedies. From the 1950s onwards, extremely effective drugs began to be introduced that brought about dramatic improvements in previously intractable conditions. As a psychiatrist practising throughout this period, I can testify to the remarkable changes that ensued.

The combination of these innovations – new attitudes towards the mentally ill, powerful drugs and effective talking therapies – led to the emptying and eventual closure of many of those Victorian institutions, and the successful treatment of their patients in the community. Others who suffered from less serious disorders could also be helped to regain their equilibrium and emerge from depression and return to normal life. Whether the patient is suffering from a major psychotic illness or a minor neurosis, the prospects of recovery have never been better than they are today – and psychological medicine continues to break new ground. We do not yet understand everything there is to know about mental illness, but we continue to seek new knowledge to improve patients' well-being. One can confidently predict that further great strides will be made in the understanding of brain function during the next decade. These will undoubtedly lead to even more effective treatment.

Physical treatments

Physical treatments in the main consist of medication, though at the end of this section we will also look briefly at electro-convulsive therapy and alternative remedies.

The period after the end of the Second World War saw dramatic advances in drug development generally, which changed the face of medicine. Antibiotics and prophylactic immunization overcame many infections; ACE inhibitors and beta-blockers enabled heart failure to be treated; an understanding of hormones allowed the development of contraceptives; and a range of other new drugs gave doctors the power to help conditions where treatment had hitherto been unimaginable.

However, these improvements were more than matched by the progress achieved in psychiatric medicine. New antipsychotic and antidepressant drugs proved to be vastly more effective than the limited treatments previously available to us – to take only one example, it was amazing to witness for the first time the effect of a drug called Largactil (chlorpromazine) on very disturbed chronic schizophrenics, and to see their relief as severe symptoms of delusions, hallucinations and bizarre behaviour disappeared. There is no doubt that we now have available to us a powerful pharmacopoeia, which enables us to treat many conditions effectively.

However, we still struggle with one issue which with most patients is beyond our control: compliance. Once a drug has been prescribed, it is important that the patient takes it at the correct dosage, at the right regular intervals and for the appropriate period of time. It is stating the obvious to say that drugs will not be effective if they are not taken. Yet it is remarkable how great the non-compliance rate is: in some studies 60 per cent of patients prescribed antidepressants in outpatients departments fail to take them. Why?

Some patients have concerns about their prescription; if this is the case, they should feel able to discuss these in detail with their doctor. They have the right to express any doubts, to ask about the effects of the drug, how necessary it is to their condition, how long it will take to become effective, whether they should expect any side effects and for how long they will have to take it. It is imperative that the psychiatrist should answer all such questions fully; most patients are reassured once they have information about their medication, and are thus much more likely to take it reliably.

One of the fears that people express most often in my clinic is that they will become addicted. There is a general misunderstanding that all psychotropic drugs prescribed for mental disorders are addictive, just like the illegal drugs such as heroin and cannabis. This is not true. In the past, some of the anti-tension drugs such as Valium and Librium were prescribed extensively (mainly in the 1960s and 1970s), before it was fully understood that they could become addictive (and that they caused some severe symptoms when they were discontinued suddenly). They are now prescribed less frequently, as they have been partially replaced by improved medications; however, they still have their uses in certain conditions, as long as doctors apply strict criteria for their use and supervise their withdrawal carefully. The newer anti-tension drugs are not so addictive, and millions of patients can attest to their successful treatment over limited periods, after which they successfully ceased treatment.

Another common fear is that the drugs will not work. This can be exacerbated by the fact that occasionally it is necessary to adjust the dosage before finding the right formula for a particular patient: one always begins conservatively with the lowest dose regarded as therapeutic, increasing it slowly if needed. Occasionally, if this low initial dose seems ineffective (or, indeed, if the patient is unwilling to wait for the medication to take effect, which can take several weeks) he or she becomes impatient and concludes that the medication "doesn't work". Stopping medication abruptly is also unhelpful and may cause side effects; the dose should be tapered down gradually over several days.

Even before discussing their medication with their psychiatrist, many patients have gathered information – and prejudices – from many sources: the internet, the press, television programmes (not always balanced and often anxiety-provoking) and anecdotally from friends. Interviewers and interviewees on television and radio programmes seldom have any personal experience of medicine before the 1950s – if they did, they would have a greater understanding of the advances we have made and the role of psychotropic drugs in this revolution. They also fail to understand the nature of some conditions such as depression, which can be a symptom of several different illnesses.

This becomes clear when listening to groups of people discussing the matter, or listening to TV or radio programmes when ex-patients tell their stories and pressure groups are given air time. Too often no effort is made to identify the problems from which the interviewees are suffering: all are labelled merely as "clinical depression". Yet while patients suffering from a classical major depressive episode are likely to have a good prognosis, many of those suffering from depression from other causes have a much less encouraging outlook. Their complaints that medication "did not work" need to be viewed in the context of their whole condition.

Unfortunately it is often the patients who tend to do least well with medication who are most likely to put themselves forward for interview. They may have personality disorders with some depressive symptomology, and some are histrionic personalities who seek the attention of the medically naïve media. They may genuinely be disappointed in the failure of their doctors to prescribe a pill that can magically rebuild a psyche that (for environmental or genetic reasons) cannot cope with the stress of their lives. Nevertheless, their complaints help to perpetuate the myths about medication, especially since they are usually the most vocal.

Patients should regard such sources of information as inadequate. We return to the fact that expert and accurate diagnosis is vital, and patients should be able to rely upon their psychiatrist to prescribe the best treatment for their condition.

Antidepressants

Before the late 1950s there were no true antidepressants: we used to prescribe amphetamines for those suffering from depressive illness. These served merely as mood-boosters; patients improved for a short while but they would become more depressed when the effect of the drug wore off. The development of real antidepressant medication was a true breakthrough.

The first antidepressant drugs were known as tricyclics because of the nature of their chemical composition. Drugs usually have a brand name (the manufacturer's trade name), which starts with capital letter; I have also given the generic name of the drug in brackets. Tryptizol (amitriptyline) and Tofranil (imipramine) effectively removed symptoms of clinical depression such as depressive mood, early-morning waking, loss of libido, loss of weight and other biological symptoms. Then came Anafranil (clomipramine), which was particularly helpful in obsessional states, and Prothiaden (dothiepin) and Gamanil (lofepramine). Related to these are other antidepressants still in common use, such as Zispin (mitrazapemine).

The next group of antidepressants that were discovered were the monoamine-oxidase inhibitors, which worked by blocking a particular enzyme. They can be most effective for neurotic or atypical depression, and are prescribed sometimes alone and occasionally in combination with other antidepressants. However, they were found to have some severe side effects, so they were largely withdrawn; nowadays they are used only infrequently, in depressive illnesses that do not respond to other drugs.

The mechanism of the depressive state is a chemical imbalance in which neurotransmitters such as serotonin and/or noradrenalines drop to a lower level than normal. It is the biochemical nature of this type of depression that makes it suitable for treatment with chemicals. The newer antidepressants redress the balance rather in the same way as insulin treatment redresses the balance in the diabetic patient. The drugs increase these neurotransmitters in the brain so that they return to their normal levels and thus counter the symptoms of depression.

The third major group which are of recent development are known as the SSRIs (Selective Serotonin Re-uptake Inhibitors). The best-known of these include Prozac (fluoxetine), Seroxat (paroxetine) and Citramil (citalopram). The SSRIs work by increasing the levels serotonin in the brain. In addition to being used to treat depression, they are effective in treating anxiety, panic and obsessive compulsive symptoms. They are also being used in cases of social phobia and eating disorders. More recently, further related compounds have been used clinically, such as Efexor (venlafaxine) and Edrinax (reboxetine).

In general, these newer antidepressants are found to be extremely effective, with the advantage of having fewer side effects than the tricyclics. All drugs have some side effects, and most of these generally disappear within a few days as the body becomes used to the drug. Patients must balance these out against the benefits of the medication.

Some patients have other concerns which may be allayed: the new antidepressants, unlike the tricyclics, are not sedating, and they seldom cause great weight gain. It must be emphasized again that they are not addictive. The taking of the medication should be monitored and controlled by regular attendance at outpatients to see the psychiatrist, and there may also be help available from the community psychiatric nurse who will help to note the effects of the medication.

It is important that an adequate therapeutic dose is taken: if a high dose is required for some time, the supervising doctor may recommend that the dose is reduced slowly over a number of days to assess whether the maintenance course can be lower. If it is to be stopped, this must be done gradually. When patients discontinue their prescription prematurely without the consent of the doctor, they find that their symptoms return.

It is usually necessary to take antidepressants for about six to nine months after the symptoms have cleared. Around 80 per cent of people suffering from a major depressive illness will improve with antidepressant medication within six to nine months. However, it is an illness that recurs: 50 per cent of sufferers will experience a recurrence within five years. There is also a group of people who can be regarded as suffering from chronic depressive illness, which implies that they should be on a continual maintenance dose of antidepressants indefinitely; they must also be monitored by a psychiatrist or a member of his team.

Certain antidepressants have some anti-anxiety properties and these are used when anxiety is the most prominent presenting symptom, although there is generally some associated depression. Tryptizol (amitriptyline), a tricyclic, is a good example of an antidepressant used for sedative effect, while we have already emphasized that SSRIs such as Seroxat are also effective in this way.

Mood stabilizers

Mania can be an illness on its own, or it may be part of a manic depressive psychosis. Usually the psychiatrist will initially prescribe an antipsychotic drug to control the manic symptoms, especially hyperactivity and agitation.

The first of the antipsychotic medications were the phenothiazines, specifically Largactil (chlorpromazine), introduced in 1952. It heralded the start of the chemical revolution that has so transformed treatment. After this a large number of different phenothiazine compounds appeared, and at first we thought these drugs would cure psychotic conditions. Sadly, this was not the case, and we had to accept their limitations. However, they do effectively reduce the hyperactivity, elation and other symptoms, such as racing thoughts. They work quite quickly and may be discontinued once acute symptoms have settled.

Another useful class of drugs is the butyrophenones, especially Serenace (haloperidol), which is extensively used. Mood stabilizing drugs are used to stop mood swings – from depression to mania and back again. People usually have to take them for a long time after their symptoms have significantly improved, in order to prevent further attacks and remain well. It is possible for someone to have one episode of a manic depressive disorder and never have another; alternatively they may remain free of illness for several years before there is a recurrence. For those who suffer from more than one episode, the psychiatrist may recommend continuing treatment with lithium.

Lithium is used to combat manic high: it will usually reduce severe manic symptoms in about two weeks, though it may be a month or more before the condition is controlled. Lithium therapy can cause side effects such as a fine tremor of the hands, increased thirst, increased urination and weight gain. It is known that lithium treatment may affect the thyroid gland, and this is carefully monitored by means of blood tests.

Not all patients with recurrences of mania and/or depression benefit from lithium. Some need to be treated with other forms of medication such as anticonvulsant drugs which are also used to treat epilepsy. The two most often used in this way are carbamazepine and sodium valproate; the first is especially effective in people with very rapid changes of mood. Unwanted side effects may include drowsiness, unsteadiness, nausea and headaches. Sometimes several drugs are used in combination to treat mania.

Antipsychotic medication

Many lay people find the whole business of antipsychotic drugs to be a complicated maze: even the names of the drugs are long and difficult, and it is sometimes hard to know how they work. In principle they affect the chemical messengers in the brain known as dopamine: the drugs reduce the amount of dopamine at the ends of the nerve cells.

After chlorpromazine, the forerunner, other phenothiazines were introduced, including Stelazine (trifluoperazine). Later it was found that these could be given as long-acting drugs by injection, such as Moditen (fluphenazine). This meant that if the patient could not be relied upon to comply by taking oral medication regularly, he or she could be given an injection every few weeks instead.

Some of these neuroleptic drugs had unwanted side effects such as stiffness, muscle pain and shaking rather like that which is experienced in Parkinson's disease. Many patients complained that they felt worse when they were taking the drugs than they did when they had active symptoms of their psychotic illness: for them, the benefits did not outweigh the side effects, and they discontinued their treatment. In fact, it now seems likely that these early problems were caused by the dosage being too high.

Drugs developed subsequently include Serenace (haloperidol, already described for its use in cases of mania) and Orap (timozide, used in specific paranoias). Newer drugs include the atypical antipsychotics such as Clozaril (clozapine), Risperidol (risperidone), Zyprexa (olanzapine) and Solian (amisulpride).

Some people claim that these drugs are less likely to cause side effects; however, several of them may cause weight gain. Many of them (such as clozapine) are especially useful for dealing with the negative symptoms of schizophrenia such as lethargy, lack of motivation and feelings of flatness. However, this drug has the possible serious side effect of reducing the number of white cells in the blood and thus reducing the body's capacity to fight infection.

Quite apart from the problem of side effects, there are difficulties in getting people to comply with their treatment. In episodes of acute mania or schizophrenia, patients are often extremely reluctant to take medication. Even if they can be persuaded to comply, once they have improved they tend to discontinue it too soon. To prevent further episodes of psychotic illness, patients should continue with the treatment even when they have been feeling better for some time.

Patients may need to continue the treatment for many months, years or even the rest of their lives. This can be a daunting prospect. The antipsychotic drugs are not addictive but they do change the way a person feels. While the patient may find it hard to accept the side effects, the health professionals may feel that these are trivial when compared with the benefits accruing from the drug: clearing delusions and hallucinations and reducing the frequency of episodes of the illness. This is where family, friends and the medical team may be helpful in persuading the patient that the medication is essential. An understanding of the drug regime will help not only the patient, but also the carers, whether they are family members or medical professionals.

Anti-tension drugs

The antipsychotic drugs described above are called major tranquillizers; the anti-tension or anxiolytic drugs are called minor tranquillizers. They relieve tension and anxiety and have some hypnotic effect; they thus help to treat both anxiety and sleeplessness. Benzodiazepines such as Valium and Diazepam are not a cure for anxiety or sleeplessness but they do alleviate the symptoms. They were prescribed on a very large scale for a number of years, which led to people becoming addicted to them. As a result there was then a reaction and psychiatrists became very reluctant to prescribe them, particularly as alternative ways of dealing with sleeplessness and anxiety became available. However, they are still prescribed for acute conditions (particularly anxiety), but only for short periods and under strict controls.

Electroconvulsive therapy

There has always been a degree of controversy about ECT (or "shock" treatment as it is sometimes known); it is clearly an entirely different kind of physical treatment from medication, and many people feel that it is indeed "shocking" and invasive. In fact, ignorance about its use causes unnecessary anxiety, especially among those for whom it is prescribed. ECT has had a bad press, suffering at the hands of ill-informed TV and radio programmes and melodramatic films. It is used very rarely today, but in certain conditions it can be a useful alternative – for instance, in severe incapacitating depressive illness where there is active suicidal risk, and which does not respond to drugs, or in situations where drug treatment cannot be tolerated.

It is particularly helpful when patients cannot tolerate the side effects of standard medication, or when someone is acutely disturbed, agitated or suicidal. In these situations it can be life-saving. There is an extreme depressive disorder called Cotard's syndrome, where patients are in despair, believing that they are already dead; under this delusion they refuse to eat or drink, and thus their life is threatened. ECT can be extremely effective in these cases, where no other treatment is possible.

Usually more than one ECT is needed, and on average two to four treatments are given at weekly intervals. It may be performed as either an inpatient or outpatient procedure, but in both cases it must be carefully monitored. If it is given at the outpatient clinic, patients must be accompanied, because they may be drowsy for a variable period afterwards. Electroconvulsive therapy involves the application of a small electrical stimulus to the brain for a very short period of time. This produces some twitching of the arms or face, implying that there has been a seizure: the procedure is effective only if this occurs. However, these effects are minimized by anaesthesia, including a muscle relaxant and a sedative; the patient is unconscious when the ECT is administered and the time of the fit is measured and controlled. Patients recover as they would from any general anaesthetic.

In the UK ECT is highly regulated and given only in clinical units that are equipped to perform it. The anaesthetic is administered by a qualified anaesthetist, and the psychiatrist and other staff are fully trained to perform the therapy.

The procedure is explained to patients beforehand and given only with written consent, except in special circumstances under the regulations of the Mental Health Act. All aspects of the treatment are fully explained by the psychiatrist and discussed with the patient and relatives; often it is possible for patients to talk to someone who has previously undergone the treatment.

I once gave ECT to an 86-year-old woman who was suffering from a literally hellish depression. She believed that she was completely evil, she was without hope, she would not eat and she was in utter despair. After three ECTs she made a remarkable recovery. The treatment was so successful that when her depression recurred two years later, her two sons insisted that I give her the "wonder cure" again.

Alternative remedies

There is one other area that we need to consider: the so-called "alternative remedies". Increasingly in recent years people have turned to alternative medicine for help, including homeopathic medicine, reflexology, chiropractic, acupuncture and various Eastern mystic techniques. These vary greatly and Christians should be aware that some of them exist in grey areas between the physical, mental and spiritual, while others are simple physical treatments.

For instance, chiropractice is a physical manipulation technique, and is so close to mainstream physiotherapy (and osteopathy) that many GPs refer their patients to chiropractors. Homeopathy – in which minute amounts of substances are diluted in water until there is no identifiable trace of its presence left – has a following, though there are suggestions that its main value for patients is that practitioners take a full and detailed case history, giving patients more time to be "heard" than is usual in a consultation. However, there are GPs within the NHS who also practise homeopathy because they believe that it works.

Acupuncture, though very much an alternative therapy in this country, is part of mainstream medicine in China, and is practised in hospitals. Reiki healing and reflexology are on the boundary of the physical and mystic, and Christians should take great care when becoming involved with these philosophies, or with other forms of "spiritual" healing. It is essential that the psychiatrist knows when patients are using alternative remedies; some of them may have some involvement with the occult, and this can be an important consideration when severe mental disorder does not appear to improve.

Many of these remedies seem to rely for their beneficial results almost entirely upon the placebo effect, in which patients feel better because they believe that something is being done for them. However, one increasingly popular alternative remedy is the use of herbal medicine, and unlike the others, it has very definite and measurable effects. People often think that if something is called "herbal" or "natural", it cannot be harmful. This is not so. Many of our most potent drugs have their origins in plants and herbs, though often we have learned to mimic their effect by recreating their chemical composition.

Herbal remedies can be very powerful. One commonly used herb is St John's wort (Hypericum perforatum). This is used a great deal in Germany, and great claims have been made for its efficacy in relieving mild to moderate depression. This is excellent if it works for a particular patient; however, it should not be used in combination with other remedies, especially with prescribed medication, as it may interact with other drugs. The psychiatrist should always be told if a patient is taking any other remedy at all.

Psychological treatments

Psychotherapy in general is a very powerful form of treatment: it can change ingrained patterns of behaviour and help people to grow and mature. Christians often oppose it because they are afraid that their "free will" will be usurped, but this is not the case. No psychotherapy can change people against their will. The most it can do is return people to their best, or enable them to behave in the way they want, and thus enable them to perform to their optimum.

The vast majority of psychiatrists carry out some form of psychotherapy, and some undertake further training in order to specialize in this treatment. The Royal College of Psychiatrists has a section for psychotherapy, and constantly emphasizes the need for all psychiatrists to receive basic training in this discipline. The famous psychiatrist Sir Dennis Hill once said that psychotherapy was the *sine qua non* of all psychiatrists.

There are two main kinds of psychological treatment: cognitive behaviour therapy and psychodynamic therapy.

Cognitive behaviour therapy

This is one of the new psychotherapy techniques that have proved particularly effective in the treatment of anxiety, panic and depression. In the most severe cases of psychosis it is usually used as an adjunct to the drug therapy described above; however, in milder cases there is overwhelming evidence that it is very effective on its own.

During episodes of illness, psychological support from the psychiatrist or other members of the team is essential: talking treatments are a special form of this, with the aim of effecting changes in a person's thoughts and feelings as well as providing general care and support. Cognitive behaviour therapy (CBT) helps people identify and challenge the way they think: for instance, recurring thoughts such as "I am a bad person" or "I will fail at anything I try" can become self-fulfilling prophecies.

CBT focuses on how people think about a situation (cognition) and what they do about it (behaviour). It aims to make them aware that the way they think and feel affects their actions. By helping them change how they think and feel, CBT allows them to try out new and more productive behaviours. If you undertake a course of CBT you may be asked about your childhood experiences, but most of the focus is on the "here and now" – the way you see and do things at present.

The psychiatrist may carry out the CBT himself, or he may refer the patient to a clinical psychologist, a community psychiatric nurse or a nurse therapist who has been trained in the technique.

Treatment using CBT involves identifying and then challenging extreme and unhelpful thoughts, and planning ways to overcome the reduced activity and unhelpful behaviour that may be a part of depression and anxiety. It does this by asking questions about thought processes and responses to events, and providing suggestions and information to help people make changes in the way they feel and react.

CBT treatment can be given on an individual or a group basis; there is evidence that CBT principles can be taught to self-help groups, and that people can have considerable success in improving their condition through such groups. Dr Chris Williams and his colleagues have described this form of treatment, specifically as applied to the Christian, in their practical book, *I'm Not Supposed to Feel Like This*.[1] NICE (The National Institute for Clinical Excellence) has also produced booklets which are particularly helpful to people needing guidance in dealing with depression,[2] anxiety and panic.[3] They are aids to patients, families, carers and the public.

For the Christian, there is usually a great deal of support available through the church fellowship if it is understanding and informed. Once the initial depression and anxiety has been improved by means of medication, CBT and psychotherapy, the way is clear for more active CBT, and here scripture can be very helpful. The patient can be helped to meditate on relevant scriptures such as:

> *Cast all your anxiety upon him, because he cares for you.*
> 1 Peter 5:7

> *I will never leave you or forsake you.*
> Hebrews 13:5

Do not fear, for I have redeemed you;
 I have called you by name, you are mine.

Isaiah 43:1

No one will snatch them out of my hand.

John 10:28

One may well ask why we should need a psychiatrist when we have God's love and care, but we have already considered this. We have to recognize that Christians can and do "crack up", and that pastors, counsellors and others can only do so much. There is no place for the amateur psychiatrist (though there may be one for the amateur counsellor, or at least befriender). It is necessary to seek professional help for psychiatric problems – and that help is a gift of God for our solace and healing.

The Psalms can be of particular help to the Christian who is recovering from mental illness. The psalmist has experienced most of the emotions and faced most of the problems we encounter. A prayerful and meditative reading of the Psalms can bring comfort and hope to the Christian.

For God alone my soul waits in silence,
 for my hope is from him.
He alone is my rock and my salvation,
 my fortress; I shall not be shaken.
On God rests my deliverance and my honour;
 my mighty rock, my refuge is in God.
Trust him at all times, O people;
 pour out your heart before him;
 God is a refuge for us.

Psalm 62:5-8

Psychodynamic therapy

This therapy has been in vogue for over a century, and was developed from the psychoanalytic theories of Freud and Jung. In it, the therapist tries to identify unhelpful patterns of behaviour that are linked with unconscious conflicts and defence mechanisms, which are used repeatedly by the patient in his or her relationships with others.

The fundamental principle is that disturbed behaviour in the present has a link with some damaging experiences in the past. The patient may have suffered some emotional hurt but repressed it and pushed it deep into the unconscious. However, at times of stress it is no longer possible to keep the damaged emotions closed off; the person regresses, re-experiences and reacts to the pain, which affects their behaviour.

For example, we have seen how often a disrupted family life – especially continual conflict between the parents – can lead to mental scarring for young people. One middle-aged woman told me recently that she had never felt adequate or confident since her father walked out on the family when she was aged eight. Around that time she developed a skin lesion which had persisted ever since; she also realized that her distress at the separation had marred her life. She had become extremely sensitive – to the point of being paranoid – and she had never been able to sustain relationships.

Psychodynamic therapy sessions occur regularly, usually once a week for an hour. In these sessions patients often reveal some of their deepest thoughts and feelings; they may abreact (act out) to these with powerful emotional outbursts, which often are very cathartic and lead to healing. By examining the past hurts that are revealed in this way, people find that they are able to accept and understand them, and change the way they behave in response to them. Their symptoms of anxiety and depression are relieved and they become more effective in their relationships.

The therapy can be performed with individuals or in groups. The process may continue for a year or two, but there is a form of brief psychotherapy that focuses on specific aims over about six months, and this can also be quite effective.

I once treated a young man of twenty who was suicidal and refused to take any medication. He had been about to marry, with the wedding planned and a house ready for them to move in to, when his fiancée met someone else and jilted him. He was in despair, and often ended our therapy sessions by saying, "But I shall kill myself anyway." At the end of a two-year course of psychotherapy he made a full recovery. As he was leaving after his final session, he turned to me and said, "You've been like a surgeon. You cut all the bad bits out and put me together again." Psychotherapy does work.

Supportive psychotherapy

Supportive or superficial psychotherapy, although it does not work at such a deep level, should not be disregarded. Most people being treated with medication also need supportive psychotherapy as an adjunct to that treatment, and people with less severe problems, such as mild anxiety, depression, guilt and fear, can be treated with supportive psychotherapy alone. This form of therapy does not attempt to make gross changes to behaviour patterns; however, by giving patients the opportunity to share their problems and to abreact to certain events in their lives, it often has a very beneficial effect. Many well-known figures in important posts have found that supportive psychotherapy has helped them to meet the challenges of their responsibilities.

Other techniques

There are other helpful techniques associated with the main psychological therapies. Counselling is now a very common form of treatment – indeed, one could say that we are in the midst of an epidemic of counselling. Some counsellors are well trained, but others are less so; it is wise to examine the qualifications of anyone setting themselves up to be a counsellor. Many counsellors specialize in certain areas such as relationship and marital counselling, or bereavement counselling. Most of these operate from a secular world-view, though there are now centres of training for Christian counsellors.

As an addition to the "talking cures" – especially cognitive behaviour therapy – many people find it useful to learn some relaxation techniques, which can be taught by nurse therapists. Relaxation can also be self-taught, from CDs, videos or DVDs; these vary in competence but can be very helpful. Most of these techniques involve the progressive relaxation of groups of muscles around the body; the exercises for controlling breathing are especially helpful to people who suffer from hyperventilation when anxious.

This chapter has given a glimpse of the therapies that are available in psychiatry today, both physical and psychological. Each has its limitations, but we must emphasize that these treatments have been shown to be effective. We have also noted their side effects, for no active therapeutic intervention is possible without potential side effects. We have also emphasized that it is important to ensure that therapists are adequately qualified and fully trained. Compliance with treatment is essential for a successful outcome.

All these therapies are not simply man-made but God-given, and there is always a missing factor in all healing which God alone fills. We turn to this in the following chapters.

Notes

1 C. Williams, P. Richards and I. Whitton, *I'm Not Supposed to Feel Like This* – a Christian self-help guide to depression and anxiety (London: Hodder & Stoughton, 2002).

2 NHS National Institute for Clinical Excellence, *The Treatment of Depression in Adults – Understanding the NICE Guidelines*, 2004.

3 NHS National Institute for Clinical Excellence, *The Management of Panic Disorder and Generalised Anxiety Disorder In Adults – Understanding the NICE Guidelines*, 2004.

8

THERAPIST AND PASTOR

When Christians say, "I want a Christian psychiatrist", what they are really saying is that they want both mental and spiritual support and healing; they want a combination of a therapist and a pastor. They recognize that they need medical intervention through medication and psychotherapy, but they also want emotional reassurance and spiritual guidance: they know that their healing must encompass their whole selves, mind, body and spirit.

The parable of the Good Samaritan (Luke 10:29-37) provides us with a useful model for support relationships. A man was on a journey from Jerusalem to Jericho when he was set upon by thieves, beaten and left "half dead". Two people were instrumental in securing his recovery. The Samaritan traveller took care of his most urgent needs and provided his primary care; then he handed over to the innkeeper, who supported the patient during his recovery and rehabilitation until he was able to take up his normal life again. In this situation, each carer has a role to play at the appropriate time.

We can imagine a similar division of labour between the medical team and the Christian's church minister. Ideally, each should be aware of the other (though of course if the patient wishes to keep secret his or her referral to a psychiatrist, this confidentiality must be respected at all costs). If necessary, and with the permission of the patient, the two may confer about the best way in which the church could offer support.

Of course, the roles of the psychiatrist and minister are different. As a psychiatrist I willingly submit to the superior and much wider role of the minister – he is the ambassador of Jesus Christ, bringing the message of salvation and healing to people through God's word. I am merely a medical practitioner specializing in the field of diagnosis and treatment of mental disorders. We have explored the role of the psychiatrist in some detail. What of the role of the pastor?

The failure of pastoral care

Christians in our country are in a minority. Where once the vast majority of the population attended church regularly, now only a small proportion of people genuinely feel that they are part of a worshipping community. I do not propose to examine the possible causes of the decline in churchgoing in Great Britain; I merely remark on it in passing as part of the increasing fragmentation of society, where families may be dispersed around the country, and there are fewer community ties or communal activities. The result is that far fewer people identify with their local community in any way; many work long hours and their leisure time may be spent largely alone in front of the television or computer.

Many people – not only those who suffer from mental illness – find themselves suffering increasingly from social isolation, with few social interactions even of the most casual kind. Where once they might have confided in their friends or the church minister, they find themselves alone with their worries. Frequently, the only trusted and authoritative figure they know is their GP. Mild conditions, and even depressive tendencies in the healthy, which could be improved with the right social support, may get worse in these situations. Too often our churches are empty and our clinics are full.

Even among Christians we find a similar reluctance to confide in the pastor. Why should that be? The answer is that with certain notable and honourable exceptions, there is something wrong with pastoral care today.

The term "pastoral care" is a description of the relationship of the minister and his congregation, likening it to that of a shepherd and his flock. The shepherd knows each member of his flock individually; he cares for them, guides them to the food and water they need, protects them from danger, binds up their wounds and supports their healing. The minister aims to provide all this for the congregation by building relationships. His work is the ministry of God's word, bringing the good news of salvation through Christ to each individual by being the ambassador of Jesus Christ. He helps them to grow and supports them in times of trouble. He tries to bring people into a right relationship with God through fellowship with Christ. By means of prayer, the sacraments and preaching the gospel, he aims to bring his people to holiness via repentance, forgiveness and God's grace.

Many ministers do all these things with devotion and care. However, I wish that ministers in general were more effective in dealing with people, and specifically with their problems. I once read some reflections on the subject written by a group of young pastors. The first, who was known as a powerful preacher, wrote, "I have been in my church for five years, but not one member has come to me with a problem." Another said, "We use the label of pastoral care to describe the close relationship of a minister and his people, yet it has become merely a method to encourage attendance at services – or to give some advice on specific circumstances – or even an opportunity to call and chat about the superficialities of life." The third wrote, "In the increasing complexity of modern life, difficulties arise in our traditional methods of pastoral care. The oh-so-nice visits, monopolized by gossip and trivial talk, are a pure waste of time. We have failed to break through to the real fears and tragedies of the souls in our care."

This is surely the basis of all therapy: to "break through to the real fears and tragedies" in people's lives. The term "pastoral care" fails to describe the real depth and intimacy of what this relationship should be. It is the part of a minister's work that gives him the opportunity to come into close relationship with his people, to meet them in the crises of their lives – in anxiety, loss, depression or doubt. Like Ezekiel, who sat down with the exiles by the river of Chebar (Ezekiel 1:1) as they wept by the rivers of Babylon (Psalm 137:1), we can help and heal simply being beside them and listening to them with empathy. It is at such times that people ask questions, reveal their deepest selves and seek for change. This is the opportunity to help them to growth, health and salvation.

Pastoral care could become more effective if it embraced some of the insights of psychology, and indeed, some of the techniques of modern psychiatry. In broad terms one could say that the whole church should be seeking for effective methods of ministering to people in need, without compromising its heritage – and without neglecting the scientific advances of modern psychology. Psychotherapy deals with emotions and mental conditions and the relationships between people. It can help the spiritual director who is attempting to support church members who suffer from mental disorders. It can also help the pastor who is trying to deal with the emotional issues of relationships between fellow Christians, and the spiritual issues of the relationships between them and God.

How counselling works

The psychiatrist, psychotherapist or counsellor who is working with patients tries to convey understanding, sympathy, confidence, genuine concern and an ability to help. Once patients are sufficiently confident in the doctor's ability and care, they can pour out their fears and admit to other emotions which may be troubling them, such as depression, hostility, anger and guilt. It is as they do this that the doctor uses a skilful blend of authoritative persuasion, suggestion and directive advice, coupled with supportive reassurance, non-directive sympathetic listening and understanding, to help them to move forward. This atmosphere of trust underlies all the "talking therapies", from deep psychotherapy to the most superficial counselling, and may be used for everything from severe anxiety states and reactive depression, to phobic states and even obsessive compulsive disorders.

In some cases patients will learn to analyze their thoughts and feelings and adapt their behaviour and responses to stimuli; in some they will learn to come to terms with their past; sometimes they grow in strength and maturity and feel able to make changes in their lives; sometimes they manage to develop coping strategies that enable them to resist, say, a tendency to anxiety or depression. All of these activities are possible with a suitably supportive counsellor.

Skilled pastors will be able to help members of their congregation in a similar way. As we have noted earlier, there are many individuals who find that they naturally "counsel" their friends in an informal manner, because they instinctively adopt many of the techniques outlined above, especially sympathetic listening and questioning. Pastors who take an intelligent interest in psychotherapeutic techniques can enhance this practice, while always proceeding with caution and carefully observing the boundaries between such pastoral counselling and the need for professional psychiatric treatment.

There are some features of counselling practice that are common to both psychiatrists and to skilled lay counsellors like pastors.

Contract

All therapists must be aware of the danger of taking on too much too soon. It is unfair to enter into a therapeutic relationship if there is a chance that you will not be there to give your time and take the trouble to build up the necessary relationship. If this is likely to be the case, it is better to pass the individual to another therapist.

Both psychiatrist and pastor, if they are trying to work with an individual, are well advised to make a "contract" with them. This includes an agreement about where, when, how often and for how long the interviews will last. The counsellor will have some idea, after the first two or three meetings, of how many interviews are likely to be necessary – and it is important to note that it may be that only one session will be necessary to identify the main issue and to settle, if not solve, that matter.

Some pastors feel uncomfortable about the idea of a "contract" – it seems to them to be too businesslike an attitude in what is essentially a caring relationship. Yet to embark on such a relationship without a clear understanding of such issues shows a lack of discretion. An insistence on saying, in effect, "there is no limit to my love," is to pretend to be more than human. It is of no help to anyone if the minister "burns out" because he has taken on too much.

I once talked to a famous minister, preacher and deeply caring pastoral leader, who said, "My door is open for my people 24/7." "That's fine," I replied, "but when do you have time for your family, for leisure, for study, preparation and prayer?" A sense of proportion and the ability to set priorities and limits are necessary if we are to be good stewards of the time and energy God has given us.

Nevertheless it is important to know that limits can and should be set. Many ministers do not take on the challenge of counselling people with mental disorders because they are fearful or ignorant of the issues. Many more are reluctant to engage pastorally with mental illness because the activity is open-ended, and they can see no end to the contact and its demands. Knowing that a contract is possible and desirable can make this seem to be more possible. We need courage to deal with people, and courage to let go.

Listening

Both pastor and psychiatrist know that listening is an essential feature of their counselling. It is listening that opens the way for people to share their problems, difficulties, feelings and ideas. Some of these thoughts and impulses may be unpleasant, but it is important that the listener resists the urge to condemn. Being non-judgmental does not mean that one is colluding or approving; merely that one is allowing the person the freedom to explore their own attitudes and thoughts in safety.

Silences are important: a good listener resists the urge to fill them with a response. If the patient is silent it may mean that they sense their own resistance to emotionally charged memories and ideas. They need time to get over this blockage or denial, in order to reveal their own true thinking. In this, non-verbal communication can be important. Psychiatrists often note how people communicate through gestures, movements and facial expressions.

Confidentiality

Confidentiality is essential. There must be no gossip; all confidences must be kept, and no facts gleaned during therapeutic sessions may be passed on to others (even doctors) without written permission from the client. It is only in an atmosphere of absolute trust that people can become willing to open their hearts.

Transference

It is essential that there is an empathetic relationship between the therapist – whether pastor or psychiatrist – and the individual. Freud coined the term "transference" to describe this special relationship between patient and psychoanalyst. Transference occurs in all therapeutic relationships, and it is of paramount importance that both parties understand this. These feelings may be warmly positive, especially towards the therapist – this is not surprising in view of the amount of time and energy that the counsellor is prepared to give to the subject.

Later, perhaps when the therapist suggests that the patient takes some active steps in self-help (or reduces the frequency of interviews), the patient may become more negative, and possibly even angry and hostile. These feelings are known as negative transference, and they do indicate growth – even though the patient is exhibiting them in resistance to demands that he or she should make choices and move towards rehabilitation. As long as the feelings are not too extreme, they can be dealt with in the course of the counselling process.

The counsellor, therapist or minister will also have feelings towards the individual – sometimes of warmth, and sometimes of dislike. These are legitimate responses and are known as counter-transference. These feelings may well reach proportions that enter the forbidden zones of hatred or of physical love. At that point it is imperative that the therapist or minister takes stock, discusses the situation with the individual and preferably transfers him or her to the care of another suitable person.

Discovery

Patients who have learned to trust in an empathetic relationship are more likely to be able to explore the deepest sources of their problems and anxieties. The therapist can help by observation, by noting certain key words and actions of the patient; together they can explore the issues by means of reflection, by wondering how an outward situation caused the anxiety, and what was happening to the patient when it first occurred. The counsellor may help by sensitively suggesting some known causes of anxiety – such as a threat to oneself, a relationship or a possession; conflict with another person such as a parent, sibling, friend or fellow church member; or a fear of something specific. There may be some deep inner need for something: survival, security, sex, self-fulfilment, self-esteem or a sense of identity. After identifying the cause the next crucial step is towards resolution or restoration: no amount of understanding will help unless it leads on to action.

Having discovered the cause of the anxiety or depression, the patient must be encouraged to do something about it – to reduce or eliminate it so that it ceases to affect their life, or else, if it cannot be eliminated, to learn how to cope. It is important to recognize that courage does not consist of the absence of fear and anxiety, but of the capacity to move on with life even when one is afraid. Sometimes nothing much can be done about the source of anxiety, and all the person can do is choose whether to stand still or to move on in pain and doubt. Sometimes the only role of the counsellor is to provide a calm, warm, caring, understanding source of support. Often when I have been dealing with patients who are paralysed with depression, the only thing I have been able to say is, "Hold on."

Termination

If the therapy goes on for too long, this may be a sign that the patient is resistant to dealing with the problems, refusing to change and mature. There is a risk of them becoming dependent on the counsellor, especially if no contract has set an end to the counselling period. It is easier, of course, for the psychiatrist, who is in a professional and medical relationship with the patient, to terminate it. The pastor must find a way of ending the sessions – perhaps by saying, "I have been seeing you for this amount of time... now it is time for you to grow" and reducing the frequency of visits. There may be several responses: some individuals will be angry; some will produce new problems to engage the pastor's attention; some will threaten suicide (this needs courage to resist, but is a sign that the patient should be referred for professional help); others will find fault with the therapist or minister and stop attending. Both psychiatrists and pastors will be familiar with all these moves, and most will have met individuals who become addicted to being counselled. Such people have often done the rounds of the senior pastor, the junior pastor and any leader or counsellor prepared to listen.

Working together

Some Christians find it difficult to accept that there may be any links between psychotherapy and pastoral care. They believe that psychotherapy is secular, while Christianity is spiritual, and that in linking them, psychiatry would cease to be a scientific enterprise while pastoral care would become diluted and secularized. Of course, the latter is a threat, especially if the minister focuses his attention exclusively on psychotherapeutic techniques, neglects the practice of his faith and ceases to depend on prayer and the guidance of the Holy Spirit. If the pastor's theology is weak, and he overemphasizes the importance of psychology, his pastoral care will be mere humanism with a little religious colouring.

This was Archbishop Carey's complaint regarding his clergy in a lecture he gave to evangelists in Europe. He shared his anxiety that they increasingly preached secular counselling from the pulpit rather than the healing, saving gift of the grace of God.

True pastoral care allows the minister to share in the crises of people's lives and to create an atmosphere of acceptance that is conducive to trust, including trust in God at the centre of the relationship. This kind of care can be enhanced by learning some of the lessons of psychotherapy and discovering how to help people to reveal their weaknesses and their needs, to learn to manage their anxieties, and to find hope and faith along the way.

Similarly, the psychiatrist knows that when dealing with

Christian patients it is important to be able to utilize an understanding of the spiritual issues; how else could a psychotherapist understand the despair of the depressed man who says that his greatest pain lies in being unable to pray?

However, both pastor and psychiatrist are ill advised to enter into debates about faith as a form of psychological or religious discussion. Patients may be doing this merely to avoid talking about themselves and their real problems, and attempting to draw the therapist's attention away from these into a mutually interesting but essentially neutral topic. This kind of reference to their religious problems may be merely an indication of resistance to facing their true emotional problems and contemplating the necessity of change.

It is important for the pastor and the psychiatrist to be able to refer to each other in appropriate cases. The Christian who seeks help from either should be prepared to cooperate with them; but at the same time, the therapist should understand that he must not open wounds he cannot help to close. One danger is that patients in the course of therapy realize that they have deeper problems than they ever thought they would have to face. As a result they may become despondent and even suicidal. If this occurs, they must be carefully watched and appropriate action taken.

In this situation, the pastor must recognize his limitations; if the patient has problems that are too deep for him to deal with (such as mental trauma, deep-rooted depression or anxiety) he should encourage the patient to see a GP with the aim of referral to a psychiatrist. Obvious physical symptoms such as weight loss and insomnia, or significant psychotic symptoms such as delusions and hallucinations,   suicidal   thoughts,   drowsiness, disorientation or thought disorders, are all warning signs.

As an aside, pastors should also beware of taking on patients for whom simple counselling is never going to be sufficient. Some of these are people who have sought help from many agencies without success, or who show marked features of a personality disorder, being extremely histrionic and manipulative, or being aggressive with a tendency to violence. These are also patients who should be passed on to the medical profession.

When either the pastor or the psychiatrist is assessing a person, they should be able to tell whether they are competent to deal with that person and their problem. It may be that the psychiatrist, in his turn, interviews a Christian patient and decides that the problem is not psychological at all, but clearly a spiritual issue. In that case he will be right in referring the patient to the pastor who has expertise in that area.

I have emphasized the power of modern psychiatric treatments, including psychotherapy. However, I fully accept that there are limits to what psychiatry can do. Sigmund Freud, the father of modern psychotherapy, recognised this; he saw that even after a long period of successful psychoanalysis, when all distressing symptoms had disappeared, patients often still remained unhappy. He said that this was because the "human predicament" remained. Carl Jung stated even more clearly in his book *Modern Man in Search of a Soul*,

> *People from all the civilised nations of the earth have visited me. It is safe to say that all of them fell ill because they had lost that which all the living religions of the age had given their followers, and none had been really healed unless they regained their religious outlook.* [1]

I would be more specific, and instead of saying "their religious outlook" I would say "their Christian faith".

Spiritual counselling

When we are counselling the Christian who is suffering from anxiety or depression, at first we may be able to say no more than the words we mentioned above, "Hold on." It often helps them to know that people are praying for them, and to receive assurances that their struggles will succeed in time and the black moods will pass. Lady Julian of Norwich wrote much the same thing in her fourteenth-century book, *The Cloud of Unknowing*: "All shall be well, and all manner of things shall be well."

When we turn to the scriptures with counselling in mind, it is remarkable how much helpful advice we find. There is a great deal of specific guidance that encourages the victim of anxiety to focus on those thoughts and activities which directly reduce their anxious state. Philippians 4 is a rich source of this.

Rejoice

"Rejoice in the Lord always; again I say, Rejoice" (Philippians 4:4). The command is repeated twice: even when we are anxious, as Christians we can rejoice because of Jesus' promise that he will never leave us nor forsake us (Hebrews 13:5), and will not allow anyone to snatch us out of his hands (John 10:28). With this knowledge we can hold on and trust that he is our peace; he will come again to take believers into the place he has prepared for us in heaven (John 14:1, 3, 18, 27). Focusing on these promises can help us when our thoughts tend to be troubled or fearful.

Forbear

"Let your forbearing spirit be known to all" (Philippians 4:5, RSV). There is no strict equivalent to the Greek word translated as "forbearing". It means gentleness, graciousness, consideration and kindness – qualities that do not come naturally to any of us. They come with God's grace when he changes us and we are prepared to accept the power of his Holy Spirit work in us. When that happens we lose the negative, condemning attitudes that make us demand our rights, and lead us to anger and anxiety. A gracious, forbearing attitude relaxes our fears.

Pray

"Do not worry about anything, but in everything by prayer and supplication with thanksgiving let your requests be made known to God. And the peace of God, which surpasses all understanding, will guard your hearts and minds in Christ Jesus" (Philippians 4:6). This verse gives us several instructions about prayer in times of anxiety. Such prayer should be specific, including precise petitions; it should include thanksgiving for divine goodness and should be accompanied by an acceptance that supernatural peace is the gift that will follow.

I firmly believe that prayer is a major cure for anxiety – but it is a cure available only to believers. How can you pray to a God you do not believe in? St Paul asked a similar question of the Athenians.

Think

"Finally, beloved, whatever is true, whatever is honourable, whatever is just, whatever is pure, whatever is pleasing, whatever is commendable, if there is any excellence and if there is anything worthy of praise, think about these things" (Philippians 4:8). Anxiety arises from our thinking, particularly if we are preoccupied with problems, fears, weaknesses and the anticipation of future difficulties. This beautiful verse instructs us to focus our thoughts on good things. It emphasizes the power of positive, biblically based thinking.

Act

"Keep on doing the things that you have learned and received and heard and seen in me, and the God of peace will be with you" (Philippians 4:9). Paul instructs us to put our Christian faith into action. We can think and talk too much: to be effective, our discussions must be followed by choices, decisions and actions. There is always a danger that "talking therapies" may become mere "talking". Those who go on talking and never act, also never mature, never move on and never solve their problems. This is one of the dangers of counselling, and we are shown how to avoid it.

There is always the risk that people can become addicted to therapy, especially when no tasks are faced or undertaken. In one church I helped to train a dozen or so lay counsellors, and we were able to offer deep counselling to a large number of people in a rapidly growing congregation. Many of those we saw were healed: they were delighted to accept help in uncovering the issues that were causing them distress, and overcoming them. Many of these had no recurrence of their problems. Others were helped, finished their counselling, and returned only when their problems recurred. However, about a third of the people we saw discontinued their counselling sessions with us and disappeared; all of these had shown evidence of being unwilling to confront themselves in the therapeutic situation. They preferred to go on talking to ministers, elders, church members and anyone who was willing to offer them cups of tea, sympathy and hours of listening to them talk about themselves, rather than look at their problems in depth and prepare to act to solve them.

James 1:22 tells us that our task is to do what the scriptures teach us, and not merely to listen: "But be doers of the word, and not merely hearers who deceive themselves." Perhaps there are too many armchair worriers in our churches. Even in the midst of depression and worry, anxiety can be reduced considerably when the Christian sufferer pursues this course of action. Reverting to "godly behaviour" and knowing that one is doing one's best to follow the guidance of scripture is a great comfort.

The path to healing

Christians can be greatly helped on the path towards healing by this kind of counselling. As I have said, depressives need treatment with antidepressant medication and cognitive therapy; when they begin to improve they will also begin to pray for healing, and other members of the fellowship will be giving them prayerful support. The pastor can help a great deal at this stage. Once patients are once again able to read the Bible and pray, carefully selected scriptures (notably the Book of Psalms and sections of the Epistles) will support their faith. The Bible reminds us that Christ suffered on earth like any other human being: he wept, he was angry, he suffered feelings of rejection in the garden at Gethsemane, and he felt the ultimate separation from God himself on the cross. God can identify with our feelings, and in sharing them can make them more acceptable to us. The spiritual and the psychological do overlap in the process of healing.

The role of repentance

The sorry tale of David and Bathsheba gives us a view of one aspect of spiritual healing. David sinned in several ways: he coveted another man's wife; he made her pregnant; he made several attempts to cover up his responsibility for her pregnancy by bringing her husband Uriah home and giving him the opportunity to sleep with her; and finally he connived at Uriah's death (2 Samuel 11: 2-27). He was the king, and he had the power to arrange all this so that he could bring Bathsheba into his home and make her his wife, without anyone suspecting the truth. However, he could not hide from God, who sent the prophet Nathan to deliver a message.

Nathan used a parable to reveal to David the facts he was trying to hide from himself, telling him the story of a rich man who stole the only lamb from his poor neighbour. David had no hesitation in condemning such an action – he knew right from wrong – but Nathan pointed out that he had behaved in just the same way. His intervention enabled David to admit to his crime: "I have sinned against the Lord" (2 Samuel 12:13). We can see from our reading of the Psalms the path of depression that David had to tread.

> *There is no soundness in my flesh*
> *because of your indignation;*
> *There is no health in my bones*
> *because of my sin.*
> *For my iniquities have gone over my head;*
> *they weigh like a burden too heavy for me...*
> *I am utterly spent and crushed;*
> *I groan because of the tumult of my heart.*
> Psalm 38:3, 4, 8

The problem lies deep within us, hidden and partially

repressed, causing our depression and the physical and moral symptoms of malaise. It has to be uncovered as we work through the process of disclosure.

There can be no healing without repentance; no repentance without confession; no confession without true self-awareness of the hidden thing; in David's case it was another person, Nathan, who helped him to come to this discovery. The roundabout approach of the parable allowed David to relive all the emotions bound up in his actions – the anger, self-accusation, guilt and anguish – expressing them in words enabled him to bring them into his consciousness.

Nathan's role as a prophet lifted the whole sordid affair from the realms of everyday gossip into another context: the spiritual one. In the presence of God, repentance and forgiveness have their true meaning. For full healing to occur, there is a need not only to acknowledge the unconscious conflicts, but to confess them to a forgiving God. It is this repentance and our acceptance of his love and pardon that heals us.

There are two psalms that illustrate this perfectly.

> *While I kept silence, my body wasted away*
> *through my groaning all day long;*
> *for day and night your hand was heavy upon me;*
> *my strength was dried up as by the heat of summer.*
> *Then I acknowledged my sin to you;*
> *and I did not hide my iniquity;*
> *I said, "I will confess my transgressions to the Lord",*
> *and you forgave the guilt of my sin.*
> *Therefore let all who are faithful offer prayer to you;*
> *at a time of distress, the rush of mighty waters*
> *shall not reach them.*
> *You are a hiding-place for me;*

> *you preserve me from trouble;*
> *you surround me with glad cries of deliverance.*
>
> Psalm 32:3-7

The second is subtitled "A Psalm of David, when the prophet Nathan came to him, after he had gone in to Bathsheba".

> *Have mercy on me, O God,*
> *according to your steadfast love;*
> *according to your abundant mercy*
> *blot out my transgressions.*
> *Wash me thoroughly from my iniquity,*
> *and cleanse me from my sin...*
> *Restore to me the joy of your salvation,*
> *and sustain in me a willing spirit.*
>
> Psalm 51:1–2, 12

Note that we are not saying (as so many ignorant and unkind teachers have said) that all depression is caused by sin. However, where sin is present, repentance will help us on the road to healing, once we have accepted the help that is offered us, whether it comes from a doctor, a counsellor or a prophet.

The key to healing

Spiritual direction goes further than the psychotherapy of the secular psychiatrist. Within their own framework, psychotherapy and psychoanalysis have no ultimate answers, and self-awareness and self-realization are never enough. We may identify our own underlying problems, we may make changes in our lives to remedy some of our difficulties, but in the end our "self-sufficiency" is insufficient.

This is where all the self-help books which crowd the shelves of our bookshops fail. People buy book after book that purports to tell them how to be successful, or thin, or calm, or dynamic, or happy – but none succeeds. Only a recognition of the wider framework can make us truly fulfilled – a framework that includes humankind's relationship with God, who in Christ "was reconciling the world to himself" (2 Corinthians 5:19).

The pastor who acts as a counsellor uses the insights of modern psychiatry as well as the spiritual resources of the gospel; he has the church fellowship and its sacraments to help him. Above all, he has prayer, giving access to the healing grace of Jesus. Christianity is essentially, if it is anything at all, a vital relationship with the living Christ, the one who said, "I came that they may have life, and have it abundantly" (John 10:10).

Psychotherapy with a Christian emphasis is only one form of healing ministry; there should be no competition within a church. Just as there are many gifts, but one Spirit, so there are many avenues through which healing may be accomplished: prayer, counselling, laying-on of hands. All are valid as long as they are governed by love and respect, both for the suffering person and for one another.

Above all, Christians must beware of simplistic solutions. There is no doubt that our Lord Jesus can heal instantaneously, but he also often heals slowly by degrees and through the ministry of doctors, counsellors and others. To say that Jesus heals is true, but to suggest that all the sufferer has to do is give his life to Jesus and all will be well, is misleading. I have often had to pick up the pieces after people have responded to such a suggestion only to fail because they are simply too ill to continue to walk in their Christian lives without help. We know that good, true Christians suffer from mental illness like everyone else. We can grow only by degrees in maturity in Jesus Christ.

Doctors and ministers are merely channels for the healing grace of Jesus: the Lord alone can create us anew and make us whole. Charles Wesley puts it succinctly:

> *Finish then thy new creation,*
> *Pure and spotless let us be.*
> *Let us see thy great salvation*
> *Perfectly restored in thee.*
> *Changed from glory into glory*
> *Till in Heaven we take our place,*
> *Till we cast our crowns before thee,*
> *Lost in wonder, love and praise.*

Notes

1 Carl G. Jung, *Modern Man in Search of a Soul* (New York: Harcourt Brace & World, Inc., 1933).

9

A ROLE FOR THE CHURCH

We have looked at the role of the pastor as therapist – but what about the role of the ordinary members of the church fellowship? To examine this, we need first to step back into the past.

Lessons from the past

In the early 1960s I was working as a consultant in a mental hospital with about 2,500 patients. My first impressions were not hopeful: the place was overcrowded, under-staffed, and with an atrophying rigidity in its regime. There was one ward in particular that I visited, named the "long ward" because of its long, narrow construction, which was particularly depressing. It was always kept locked, because it housed a large number of schizophrenic men with a history of past disturbance or violence. The staff did their best to keep them fed and clean, but most of them appeared beyond help: they scarcely spoke, they dribbled, urinated at will, and slopped food over their hospital clothes.

I remember initially walking in and stepping over the hunched bodies lying on the floor. My eyes strayed to the stained and dirty green walls (everything was painted green), and a rusty wire on a rusty nail, holding a broken picture which no one had dusted for years. It seemed like a symbol of the despair and hopelessness of the situation. The men here had been locked away for years and years, and it seemed that no one cared for them.

However, although they did not yet appreciate it, they were very fortunate. Largactil (chlorpromazine) was just becoming available, and I had seen with my own eyes the difference it could make. I had seen patients lose their delusions and hallucinations and become rational and civilized once more. I gathered the patients who "belonged" to me (I was their Responsible Medical Officer under the Mental Health Act), along with others from other wards, and placed them all (around thirty of them) in one ward. We made a detailed assessment and diagnosis of every case, prescribed the appropriate drugs, began to talk to the men, and watched a miracle take place.

People who had been dumb began to speak; withdrawn people became alive again. Men who had not held a knife or fork for years began to eat unaided. We opened the windows and the doors of the previously "closed" ward; we gave each man a suit of his own and clothes for leisure; we fitted the ward with a wardrobe for each man, and a rug beside each bed; we increased their activities and provided occupational therapy. After a while one or two of them asked if they might be allowed to venture into the world outside the hospital gates, and one man managed to get a job on a building site.

What was happening was the first stage in rehabilitation. Many of those patients, who had once seemed to be so helpless and hopeless, eventually were able to take their place in the world outside the high walls which had surrounded them. It was healing of a very real kind. What were the lessons we might learn from this experience?

Effective treatment

First, this transformation would not have taken place without accurate diagnosis and effective treatment. It was important that we took the time and trouble to diagnose the men's condition; we were fortunate in that at last we had a treatment that could effectively reduce their symptoms.

Care

The nursing staff had always played a crucial part in the care and management of these patients. Many of them had given loving care to these unfortunate men over many years, and their work – performed in difficult circumstances when hardly any treatment was available – cannot be measured. They were always well informed about the patients, their histories, their needs and their relationships. Together we thought about what the patients needed, what they could cope with in terms of activities, and how we could improve their lives. This level of care and consideration was vital in helping them on their way back to health.

Respect

Giving these men their own suits instead of standard, communal, hospital-issue clothing made a great difference to them. Talking to them instead of about them, asking them directly how they felt instead of consulting only the nurse in charge, and giving them increased responsibility for their own personal care and well-being: all these things showed respect for them as individuals, and enhanced their self-respect in turn.

Listening

We began to have group meetings on the ward, and patients began to talk about their feelings, their wishes, their doubts and anxieties, and even their hopes and aspirations. We listened to them and acted on their requests whenever possible. Knowing that someone was prepared to listen to them made a huge difference to the way these men viewed themselves; they were no longer written off by society and locked up away from all normal relationships. Here were people prepared to talk to them and listen to their opinions, for they were human, too.

Acceptance

Little by little, as the opening up continued, the men began to put aside their masks and exhibit the resentments and frustrations that had built up over years of incarceration: anger, jealousies and hate. We maintained an atmosphere of acceptance and understanding. They grew to understand one another and to listen to each other with the same courtesy; then they began to exhibit concern, compassion and love. Bad and good feelings alike were revealed and dealt with as the men were restored and healed.

Emotional as well as physical healing occurred as we saw growing personal relationships in a healing community. For those of us privileged to have been part of such therapeutic advances it was a profound, almost religious experience. We saw men restored to dignity, health and maturity. Most of all, it was noticeable that once the drug treatment had begun to take effect, many of the other therapeutic activities were achieved in an informal manner, by simple activities, by the nursing staff, and to a certain extent, by the patients for themselves.

A caring community?

As a result of these miraculous happenings, the gates were opened and a trickle of patients began to go outside the hospital, for shopping, for visits, and for prolonged stays with their astonished families. The trickle became a flood which continued until many of the old-style asylums were emptied. We know now that in some parts of the country this exodus occurred too quickly: the communities that received these patients were unprepared for their arrival. It meant that we had to consider another new concept, and we coined a new label, "community care".

We needed facilities for these patients who were returning home like the Prodigal Son, but too often without a father's welcome awaiting them. One part of the new Mental Health Act of 1959 had stated that local authorities should provide social workers to help them, and build new hostels and sheltered accommodation to house them. However, doubts were expressed about whether this would happen: councils had other priorities, and there is little voting potential among the mentally ill. Their medication could be continued by their hard-pressed GPs, but otherwise there was little help available. Often these patients found to their cost that the general public were fearful and unwelcoming. The stigma of mental illness meant that it was hard to find accommodation or employment, much less friendship and support. Unfortunately that stigma still remains to a significant degree in the twenty-first century.

The community did not care – not for these schizophrenic patients whose symptoms were controlled by medication, and not even for the many others who suffered from less dramatic and severe conditions, such as anxiety or depression. Mental illness was something to avoid. The churches were no better. Ignorance, fear and the stigma of mental illness were just as prevalent among Christians as among the general population. They would happily make space among the pews for a wheelchair, but there was little sympathy for the less evident disability of mental illness.

There are lessons to be learned from our experience of

healing within the hospital, and the nurturing, supporting group we had developed there. Why was the same love, care and acceptance not available within the church?

In many churches little has changed. When I am treating Christians I know that they come from a church fellowship. One of my first questions is whether the other members of that fellowship understand them; are they prepared to offer support without adding to their feelings of stigma and isolation?

Desertion

Only recently I spoke to a woman who had brought her daughter to my clinic. She told me that since her daughter had been diagnosed with a severe depressive illness, her church friends had deserted her. They no longer telephoned or visited her; they did not include her in invitations or outings; it was as if they did not want to accept that the friendship had ever existed. This kind of rejection runs entirely contrary to the spirit of loving fellowship, and denies the reality of the faith as it is preached in that church.

Prejudice

Church members not only share the fear and prejudice of the rest of the world: they often have their own set of "spiritual" prejudices. They imply that if the sufferer is not living an entirely joyful, victorious Christian life, there must be something wrong with their faith. Some Christian leaders refuse to accept that any member of their church could possibly suffer from depression, as if that "failure" would reflect on their own qualities of effective leadership and teaching. Often, members of the church reject psychiatry, drug treatment or counselling as "unspiritual";

some even going so far as to suggest that my own medical discipline is of the devil.

Indeed, in certain churches mental illness is regarded not just as a symptom of spiritual inadequacy, but as a sign of demon possession. Schizophrenia (with its hallucinations that may be auditory, so that patients report "hearing voices") is often seen as demonic, and obsessive-compulsive disorder can be seen as "oppression". Yet these conditions can be treated rapidly and effectively by medication and cognitive behaviour therapy; I am unaware of any religious teaching that demons can be exorcised by means of tablets!

Judgment

Sadly, the church historically has shown a tendency to be critical and censorious. There was a time, not too long ago, when premarital pregnancy was regarded as a cardinal sin, and a young woman in this condition (for whatever reason) would be "cut out" from the church fellowship – and this by leaders who themselves were often sexually hyperactive, to say the least. Nowadays there is a great debate within the church about homosexuality.

The issue here is not about blameless behaviour, but about the predisposition on the part of the church to label people and to treat them with insensitivity and rejection rather than understanding and empathy. No church member is perfect and no church fellowship is perfect. When a fellowship assumes that to suffer from depression, for instance, is a reflection on someone's spiritual life, this adds the burden of guilt to someone who already has enough troubles. It also makes people much less likely to admit to having such a condition, which in turn adds to the veil of secrecy and shame which surrounds mental illness.

Insensitivity

In Chapter 2 I wrote about Mrs Brown, the lady who suffered from depression, partly because of the burden of caring for her child, who had cerebral palsy. Mrs Brown was a Christian and a member of a large and flourishing church, which happened to have its meeting halls upstairs. Week after week she would struggle to carry her child up two flights of stairs to the Sunday school, and as she told me, "No one ever offered to help me." Mrs Brown was delighted when she heard that the chapel had plans to install a lift, and she was utterly cast down when the plans were scrapped. The budget had been reassigned, presumably by a committee that simply had no understanding of her plight.

She also told me that no one in that fellowship had ever offered to look after her daughter, even for half a day, to give her a break. She felt that people found it hard to contemplate having to care for a child who was unable to respond emotionally to anyone. They were unwilling to offer to spend even a couple of hours with her, because she could not smile or talk to them. No wonder Mrs Brown felt isolated from the rest of her supposedly caring church community, and even more so when she developed depression. I prescribed a course of antidepressants, and also suggested that she took a part-time job – only two afternoons a week – and used the income to pay for good nursery care for her daughter during the time she was out at work. There was almost no increase in the family income, as it was mainly spent on childcare, but the change of scenery and the adult conversation worked miracles for Mrs Brown – miracles that the church could easily have helped provide.

Why do we fail?

When I established my ward of recovering schizophrenics, I realised that I had also established a therapeutic community. In those discussion groups, where every patient was acutely aware of his own and everyone else's vulnerability, people had the honesty to confront themselves. They were willing to express their own ideas, and equally ready to accept each other's positive and negative feelings. However, when I visited my own church and others on a Sunday, I did not see the same sincerity, growth and support.

We exchanged platitudes about the weather or the sermon; we asked each other how we were, but the only acceptable answer was that we were fine. We knew little of the travail of our fellow members, and we gave each other very little support and succour. Perhaps the minister and deacons did better, but the church fellowship was little more than a social club. Too often our churches are centres of conventional religious life, terribly respectable, and demanding a certain rigid standard of behaviour based on a generally accepted Christian ethic. They are not centres where Christian love is mediated. I wondered how many others in my church felt the same way. Is the modern church filled with Christians who look and sound pure, but who are inwardly sick of themselves, their weakness and ineffectiveness, and the lack of reality in their Christian life?

This behaviour is not new. The disciples shared the life of Jesus for three years. We may sentimentalize this and choose to imagine that it must have been a beautiful experience. How wonderful to sit at the feet of the Master and hear his teaching, to share in that precious fellowship of love and care! Yet in the Gospels we have a clear account of those years, and what do we find? Disciples quarrelling among themselves about who is the most important and who will have the best seat in heaven. We hear Jesus calling Peter the devil, and telling his followers that they have not even begun to understand the ways of God or the meaning of the kingdom of heaven. We see Judas giving in to greed and resentment, and committing suicide out of remorse. Even Peter denied his Master three times. It was only by treading this difficult path of conflict, stress and tears – and by the intervention of the Holy Spirit – that they eventually came to understand the true meaning of creative healing and saving love. Why should we expect it to be any different for us?

What is love?

What do we do with our resentments, jealousies, ambitions, selfishness and sexuality in our Christian communities? Do we cover them up by straining through our own efforts to be "good" Christians? Or do we really confess them, share them with one another and find healing in the love of God? Charlotte Elliott wrote,

> *Just as I am, without one plea*
> *But that thy blood was shed for me*
> *And that thou bidd'st me come to thee*
> *O Lamb of God, I come.*

Just as I am – no humbug, no hypocrisy, no fake. We know that real love, God's love, is able to accept us sinners just as we are. Surely a church fellowship should be a place where people are free to be themselves and to find healing in the redemptive love of Christ, mediated by his body, the church.

What do we really mean by love towards one another?

Surely not a superior brand of human kindness, based on the suppression of bad feelings. One of the greatest lessons of psychiatry is the necessity to see ourselves, warts and all, before we can hope for change. Yet many Christians still live as though God loves us only when we are good, and as if we have to shut out all the evil before we can receive his love. Consequently they make it hard for themselves – and anyone else – to admit to problems, insecurities, anger or hate.

On the cross Jesus demonstrated that real love reveals sin and all the bad things deep within us; it brings it all into the light, suffers its impact and then redeems it. Christian love allows life to bring what it will, without avoidance, and it is this positive acceptance that mysteriously yet effectively changes both people and the outcome of events. One of the greatest difficulties for sinful people in a sinful world is to believe that the accepting attitude of a suffering love is more creative, and has more redemptive powers, than human control and suppression.

A healing, growing fellowship is one that changes people for the better through an accepting love. Suffering is an integral part of that process. But let us not deceive ourselves that we are the healers and that other people are the sick. We all need to share in this experience if we are to enter into real, vital, living relationships with people. We must inevitably suffer the impact of our shared humanity: our envies, hates and jealousies. If we try to help others we expose ourselves to the knowledge of our own failings, mixed motives, and sin.

A choice for the church

The Christian church today faces a stark choice. It can live for itself, closing its doors to the fouled-up lives of the damaged and despairing, and keep its hands clean, but in the process it will wither away and die, irrelevant to the world. Or it can follow Christ and build bridges to those in need, the poor and the sick, and especially the mentally ill, go out and get its hands dirty in the despairing earth of the world, and it will survive and mature and grow.

If we remain egocentric and withdrawn we will die, but if we throw ourselves into the storm of the world's needs, we will live and thrive.

God cared for us, so much that he gave his only son to die for us. He broke the barriers of time and place to enter the limited dimension of this world, to share our life on earth. The message of the gospel and the great doctrines of our faith are not theories to be argued over; they are gifts to heal and save humankind. Consequently, if our Christianity is not relevant to the real world, it is a waste of time. If the church is worth anything, it is as an extension of the incarnation, the body of Christ, the means of continuing his work in the world today.

The committed Christian is a compassionate Christian, and compassion is love in action. The convinced Christian is one who is saved by grace in a wonderful union with Jesus Christ, and is empowered to do his work.

Jesus said, "I was hungry and you gave me food, I was thirsty and you gave me something to drink, I was a stranger and you welcomed me, I was naked and you gave me clothing, I was sick and you took care of me, I was in prison and you visited me" (Matthew 25:35–36). He makes it clear that when we help others, we do it for him. We should see his face in every sufferer we meet. He stands among us with the nail prints in his hands, reminding us that he died for the neurotics, the depressives, the psychotics and all the suffering men and women, just as he did for you and me.

Households of faith

Some years ago I worked alongside a leadership team in my church to try to develop a new model for our fellowship. My vicar, the late Canon Roy Barker, was a man of great insight, and he had become aware of the inadequacy of the Bible study groups that had been running for years. These groups were run in the homes of church members, but they were constantly in flux. People would join a group and then move on, for a variety of reasons – they didn't like the coffee, or they didn't like the leader, or they didn't like the other members. Christians are remarkably good at splitting into ever-smaller groups for one reason or another.

The system we put in place, after six months of careful preparation both individually and with the church membership, was called "households of faith". Each household met at least once a month, with a convenor chosen by the leadership team. Members were invited to agree and sign a pledge to attend the same household for a minimum of two years. This had the effect of curtailing the movement from group to group: the members had to stay put; they had to suffer one another in love, and in doing so, they changed.

The groups studied scripture together, prayed and supported each other. They shared feelings and difficulties; they went through the usual upheavals of family life, births and deaths, illnesses, joys and sorrows. Remarkable events happened; ordinary life went on. The members grew to trust and rely on each other; irritations waxed and waned, and people matured and learned to live together. They became true households of faith which remained effective for years. The groups had given an opportunity for Christians to grow together.

Robert Edgar' sums up this idea, saying that such a group can be

> *A laboratory of love where persons experience the giving and receiving of acceptance, forgiveness, understanding and concern. It is a group where persons go to listen with openness and positive interest; with sacrificial involvement; with expectancy so great as to evoke the fullest capacities from each other; with patience grounded in faith in what the person may become; and without judgement but with deep care.*

We need to begin anew with a fresh honesty that declares that "all have sinned and fall short of the glory of God" (Romans 3:23). Our only hope of a renewed and resurrected church is to acknowledge our unworthiness and inadequacies, and come before the living, loving God as children in need, honestly confessing our weaknesses and perplexities, and accepting his strength, salvation, healing and leadership.

Only then can we start living together the more abundant life, the life of freedom and power in the spirit which the Lord grants to those who come to him in this way. There must be a prayer in our hearts:

> *Search me, O God, and know my heart;*
> *test me and know my thoughts.*
> *See if there is any wicked way in me,*
> *and lead me in the way everlasting.*
>
> Psalm 139:23–24

If the church becomes used to dealing with its own fellowship like this, in a spirit of humility, love and acceptance, it will be better placed to help those who suffer from mental illness. In the love that is evidenced in such households of faith, Christians will come to accept that mental illness is not caused by insufficient faith and commitment, nor by personal sin or disobedience to God.

They will see that severe mental illnesses like deep depression and schizophrenia are not due to demonic activity; great faith and claims to victory do not necessarily result in healing or deliverance. Those sufferers who are not healed are not any more sinful than those who are fortunate enough to get well. Mental illness is not merely "bad behaviour" that the victim can discard at will. In other words, compassion, understanding and love can transform our attitudes and disperse our prejudices.

Practical steps

If a church fellowship expresses its willingness to become a therapeutic community, caring for those who suffer from mental illness, how should it go about this new work?

Organize

The first thing the church should do is organize a pastoral team. Every church should be able to identify those who have gifts of encouragement, support and pastoral care. These are the people who have the key qualities: empathy, warmth, acceptance, sincerity and patience. It is important to note that such people may not necessarily be part of the leadership team, whether voluntary or paid, though the leaders should be available to offer oversight.

Such a team needs to be properly resourced with an adequate budget; time should also be allowed so that people can minister to each other, and there should be a training programme to develop listening, counselling and prayer ministry skills.

The team should be always aware of its own limitations: members should know which problems they are not equipped to tackle, and when to refer people on to other professional agencies. The pastoral team must also be warned of and take precautions to guard against abuses, such as emotional abuse, physical abuse including violence, sexual abuse such as inappropriate hugging, and spiritual abuse such as demands that people make public confessions of sins.[2]

Empower

The church that truly intends to demonstrate the love of Christ should also signal acceptance to the disabled Christians in its midst, whether those members are physically impaired or suffering from mental illness. This means empowering them to live as normal members of the church family. In the case of physical disability this may involve arranging for suitable aids – a hearing loop, a wheelchair ramp or lift. In the case of mental illness it may mean ensuring that they are supported, perhaps by a carer or a "shadow" representative, to help them participate in church decision-making or leadership roles.

Inform

One way of drawing the entire church fellowship into this caring is to make sure they have information about the nature of mental illness, dispelling the myths, fears and prejudices that abound, and enabling the members to understand a little of what life is like for sufferers. This raises the level of understanding and acceptance within the entire community.

Support

Both sufferers and carers benefit from practical and emotional support. This may take the form of regular telephone calls and visits, or offers of help. For carers who are often living under perpetual stress, the offer of specific help (for instance with shopping, DIY or cooking) can make a great difference. For sufferers who feel isolated from the rest of the community, an accompanied trip to the cinema or shops can help them to feel included.

Befriend

The easiest task, and one in which most of the fellowship is able to participate, is the simple act of befriending. So often people with mental disorders suffer from social exclusion (they may be unable to work or attend social gatherings) and personal isolation (their old friends may have deserted them or become distant). Simply being beside such people and listening to them can enable them to feel that they are no longer friendless or alone.

The qualities and activities involved are the hallmarks of a loving fellowship: tolerance, acceptance, listening, empathy, comfort without collusion, respect, reassurance and the willingness to stand alongside the sufferer. In 1999, at the launch of the Health Education Authority booklet, *Promoting Mental Health: the Role of Faith Communities*, Dr Raj Persaud said that there was a huge overlap between psychiatry and religion. "Psychiatrists are only now waking up to the fact that religion is often better at helping people cope with their suffering than psychology." At its best, a church fellowship should be the ideal place to support people.

Pray

Finally, perhaps the most effective support that the fellowship can offer is prayer, with people if they are able to pray together, or for them if their condition is such that they are unable to share in the ministry. Just knowing that others are upholding them in prayer, when they themselves can no longer find the words or feel that God is near, helps Christians to remember that that even when they feel they cannot reach God, nevertheless God can reach them. It keeps them connected to the fellowship, as part of the great web of intercession with which the church links hands in supplication to the Lord. Sometimes we can be carried by the faith of our friends.

The role of the church is to be the channel for the grace of our Lord Jesus Christ, to be a therapeutic community "plus", allowing its members to be channels of grace and healing to a sick and needy world.

Notes

1 Robert A. Edgar, *The Listening Structured Group*, Pastoral Psychology, 15 (1964), pp7–12.

2 These ideas come from C. Williams, P. Richards and I. Whitton, *I'm Not Supposed to Feel Like This – a Christian self-help guide to depression and anxiety* (London: Hodder & Stoughton, 2002).

10
HEALING AND WHOLENESS

It will be clear from the previous chapters of this book that I believe in the equal validity of all the treatments we have discussed: physical ones such as surgery and medication; psychological ones such as psychotherapy; and spiritual ones such as the laying on of hands, anointing and prayer. There is a whole spectrum of treatments which may be used individually or in combination.

Some time ago I was working on a book called *Schizophrenia: Voices in the Dark*, along with Mary Moate, who was the mother of a schizophrenic. My editor called me and said, "You're going to talk about drug treatment for schizophrenia – but what about the Christian readers who believe in divine healing?" I replied that I found no difficulty with this. I was using the drugs and the therapies which I had learned about during my long psychiatric training, and as far as I was concerned these treatments came from God. However, if the almighty God chose to intervene and heal the young man miraculously through prayer and laying on of hands, no one would be more relieved, joyful and thankful than I and Mrs Moate.

To understand the legitimacy of all these forms of healing we must return to a concept discussed in Chapter 1: that humans are made up of constituent parts – body, mind and spirit. For complete healing to be achieved, every element must be encompassed. The primary problem may be physical, mental or spiritual, but in almost every case one element will affect the others to some degree.

A striking example was a man called John, who was a highly successful businessman and an admirable Christian. John had suffered from chest problems for many years. Whenever he had an increase in breathlessness he would find that he was unable to do as much physically as he would have liked, and this limitation of his physical activity made him psychologically dejected to the extent that he would suffer from clinical depression. At the same time his depression would affect him spiritually, so that he felt unable to pray or read the Bible.

To help John we needed to work on all three elements: we treated his breathing problems; we provided him with antidepressant medication and psychotherapy; and we prayed with him and for him and supported him with our love and care. He usually recovered in a very short time. His chest would clear, his depression lifted and he would recover his ability to worship God.

This serves to illustrate the importance of a holistic approach. Body, mind and spirit are interrelated and we need to have regard for all three when we are involved in healing.

A sense of self

When we think about the relationships of these three elements, we necessarily come up against the limitations of science. Scientific, medical and pharmaceutical advances have shed a great deal of light in my own area of medicine – psychiatry – but they confine themselves to the areas of body and mind. The spirit is not yet a part of scientific investigation. Scientists admit that thus far they have not successfully addressed the key question of identity. They cannot help to answer the questions, "Who am I?", or "Who and what is the self?"

We know that the body is our outer garment: it is the

way people recognize us, by our features or our walk or our voice. It is a part of who we are. Certainly the world makes a great fuss of it. Cosmetic manufacturers spend millions of pounds on research, development and on advertising products to make faces look beautiful – as if physical appearances were the most important thing in relationships. They manage to convince a great many people of this, who then spend more money on buying the products they hope will make them look attractive. In this view of the world, personality seems unimportant.

On the other hand, the church historically has taken rather a dim view of the body (mainly, it must be said, in relationship to sex and a particularly narrow view of sin). To balance this rather negative approach we need to remind ourselves that our bodies were made by God. Nowadays when we see amazing pictures of a foetus in the womb, we can only say with the psalmist,

> For it was you who formed my inward parts;
>   you knit me together in my mother's womb.
> I praise you, for I am fearfully and wonderfully made...
> My frame was not hidden from you,
>   when I was being made in secret.
>
> Psalm 139:13–15

In verse 16 we read, "In your book were written all the days that were formed for me." That book has been partially opened for us with the discovery of DNA and the beginnings of understanding our basic structure – and it tells us yet again that each of us is unique. I am not suggesting that science will enable us to understand all the secrets of life: there is more to us than that. Paul says, "Do you not know that you are God's temple and that God's Spirit dwells in you?" (1 Corinthians 3:16).

Brain or mind?

Tied up in the question, "Who am I?" or "What is the self?" is the matter of the difference between brain and mind. What is the essential "me"?

When the artist Susan Aldworth had to undergo a diagnostic brain scan, she was fully conscious throughout the procedure. She was able to watch the monitor as the machine displayed images of the inside of her brain. She was seeing, thinking and feeling – activities we ascribe to our mind – and looking inside her own head as she did so. This inspired her to create a work of art around the pictures created by the scanner. "Where is the 'me' in all this?" she asks. "You can look into my brain, but you will not find me. I am both in my head and out of my brain. I was seeing all this and thinking all this, because of the very thing I was looking at." Her experience of using her brain to watch itself at work illustrates the paradoxical relationship between brain and mind.

We know that the brain is merely a physical organ, though admittedly we do not know as much about it as we do about the kidneys or the liver. Yet its activity produces a process we call thinking, quite unlike the process of cleansing toxins from our blood or producing urine. It produces awareness, a sense of self. It consists of "thinking flesh".

Mind or spirit?

There is yet another layer to this conundrum. Scientists who study the brain have no problem with agreeing that what we call "mind" is a way of describing this indefinable thing we call consciousness, awareness, or a sense of self. Yet Christians insist that there is something more than mere personality – we believe that there is also something called the soul or spirit. But is it more than just a function of the mind?

It is rather like our habit of attributing emotions to the heart. For anniversaries and on Valentine's Day people buy cards which generally bear a picture of a large, red, stylized heart shape – and perhaps the words, "I love you with all my heart." Yet the heart has no feeling: it is merely a pump. It might be more accurate to say "I love you with all my hypothalamus" (the organ that provides a range of relevant hormones) though it sounds rather less romantic! Yet no one denies the reality and the importance of emotion in making us who we are.

Neuropsychiatrists have recently pointed out that they have been able to identify in the brain areas that they call "God centres". The temporal lobes (the side lobes of the brain) seem to be involved when people have mystical or spiritual experiences – such as a sense of mystical unity, out-of-body experiences or religious feelings. Yet the fact that the brain is involved does not mean that there is no soul. The brain responds to both external and internal stimuli, so it could equally be stimulated by genuine spiritual activity.

Even Dr Susan Blackmore, a psychologist who has done extensive research, says that there could be more to consciousness than can be accounted for merely by looking at brain chemistry. Other scientists (such as Professor Susan Greenfield of Oxford University) say that the mind, as a personalized brain, will inevitably die with the brain at death – yet agree that there may be an imperishable part that will survive.

Science demonstrates that all our experiences are grounded in the physical state of our brain – and there is every reason to expect that the tremendous scientific advances of recent years will be multiplied over the next decade or so. Yet it still falls short of explaining the first person, the inner world of subjective awareness, the whole of the private "me".

A longing for God

It has long been recognized that there are three levels of consciousness: the conscious mind, the subconscious and the unconscious. We know that feelings, thoughts, impulses and conflicts can be repressed from the conscious to the subconscious, and beyond to the unconscious, at which depth we are almost totally unaware of them. At this level they are no longer retrievable except through dreams and deep psychotherapy. If there is damage to the psyche, evidenced by psychological symptoms, this repressed material must be dealt with before complete healing can occur.

However, there is one specific feeling that is particularly relevant to this discussion. We see in modern life an extensive unease that seems to be embedded deep in the unconscious mind. Even the most self-satisfied individual will occasionally admit to such feelings. People are constantly trying to fill this void.

They seek to ease their loneliness and longing for union by engaging in relationships of furious intensity – yet they lack commitment. They take their stresses and strains to counsellors and therapists, thinking that they can learn to live with them correctly if only they relax enough – yet they refuse to face up to their own real problems. They distract their attention from their feelings by a storm of busyness at work, or by frenetic indulgence in fitness regimes – which usually fail to satisfy. They try to kill their inner longings by dulling their awareness with tranquillizers, or by a host of behavioural sedatives which they falsely call recreation. I say "falsely", because true recreation, like true rest, leaves us with greater energy and clearer awareness; when we narcotize ourselves with drink or drugs we cloud our outlook and depress our energies.

While this fundamental unease remains unfulfilled, the individual remains spiritually disordered and diseased. As Christians who are involved in healing, whether professionally or pastorally, we need to refrain from labelling this unconscious unease as pathological, especially when it emerges into awareness. In the absence of a clearly definable disorder, it is destructive to describe this unease as an illness and regard it as something that must be remedied. On the contrary, it is the one pain we are not meant to assuage. The psalmist recognized it: "As a deer longs for flowing streams, so my soul longs for you, O God. My soul thirsts for God, for the living God" (Psalm 42:1–2).

If we allow this awareness to emerge into the light, we will reveal a longing for God – the "God-shaped space" described by St Augustine, which only God can fill. As Christian healers we need to be alert and prepared to meet people who have arrived at this point of awareness, who are beginning to long for salvation and healing. We can help to fill the void, heal the scars and restore wholeness of body, mind and spirit, by introducing them to the healing touch of the Lord Jesus.

Wholeness and holiness

Healing means wholeness; wholeness requires salvation; and salvation is the way to holiness. These concepts are linked at every level, both theologically and linguistically. In Welsh the word for health, *iechydwraeth* is close to the word for salvation, *iachawdwriaeth*. The Old English word *hal*, meaning whole, gives us our words health and holy.

Holiness is not an optional extra for the Christian. It is

one of God's imperatives: "You shall be holy, for I am holy" (Leviticus 11:45). The process of becoming holy is called "sanctification", and it is not a word that is often heard nowadays. It has not been on the Christian agenda for years, and there is a deathly silence on the subject from our pulpits. Yet holiness is the pinnacle of salvation and healing. It is the aim of all Christians; sanctification is a process of growth and maturing.

To many Christians "sanctification" conjures up the image of a restricted, limited, joyless life; a man or woman dressed in black, with a miserable face and a sanctimonious manner, saying "No" to everything, and pointing out other people's shortcomings. How did we allow the word to become so debased?

Holiness is positive. It is the glory of the heart of God placed within the hearts of humankind. Sanctification means being restored to the glory of God, making us what we are meant to be: the jewel in the crown of God's creation. The jewel is multifaceted, gleaming with the qualities that Paul described as the fruits of the spirit: "love, joy, peace, patience, kindness, generosity, faithfulness, gentleness and self-control" (Galatians 5:22).

Christ in us

It is not enough that we hear the word of God and obey it. It is necessary that we accept Jesus into our lives in the deepest sense, so that the word of God can become incarnate in our lives.

> *Jesus, take me as I am,*
> *I can come no other way;*
> *Take me deeper into you,*
> *Make my flesh-life melt away.*

Make me like a precious stone,
Crystal clear and finely honed,
Life of Jesus shining through,
Giving glory back to you.[1]

We are not to be mere spectators of the drama of salvation; we are to become involved, growing and maturing in holiness. We must grow to be more like Jesus, who lived a life without sin. It is important for us to remember that Jesus faced all the problems and temptations that we face. He suffered the same feelings and more: fear, anxiety, tension, opposition, loneliness, hatred, betrayal and desertion of friends, physical and mental pain. We cannot attain to a life of holiness, refusing to give in to temptation, by our own efforts. It is only Christ in us who helps us to gain the spiritual strength to resist: "It is no longer I who live, but it is Christ who lives in me. And the life I now live in the flesh I live by faith in the Son of God, who loved me and gave himself for me" (Galatians 2:20). In establishing a vital relationship with the living Lord, we enter into a new life as a new creation.

Growing in grace

A relationship cannot stand still: it must grow and mature with constant contact, or it will wither and die. It is no use claiming that we were saved, ten, twenty or thirty years ago, if we are doing nothing on a day-to-day basis to make that relationship grow. We grow to be like those with whom we live closely; we pick up turns of phrase, characteristic mannerisms, even underlying attitudes. It is the same with Jesus: if we want our lives to reflect his holiness we must walk with him day by day, learning his ways and loving him more.

This is the positive image of sanctification. It means

being enmeshed in Christ's love, willingly and freely setting aside our egocentricity and our narcissism, our selfish thoughts, feelings, impulses and attitudes, and replacing them with the mind of Christ. "All of us, with unveiled faces, seeing the glory of the Lord as though reflected in a mirror, are being transformed into the same image from one degree of glory to another" (2 Corinthians 3:18).

But though we are transformed by our sanctification, this does not mean that we lose our identity. We preserve our basic personalities, the shape and form of our "mind", but our spirits are changed. This affects our characters, so that our words and deeds increasingly reflect "the glory of the Lord". To be sanctified thus is to become whole, healthy and powerfully integrated with God.

God's promises

The church's silence on the subject of holiness has led to many Christians not "seeing God" as they wished. It is also responsible for the failure of countless Christians to live holy, healthy lives. When we view the sad decline in the moral and spiritual life of our nation, we have to conclude reluctantly that there is too little leadership given by the church. There is a discrepancy between our faith and our lives; between our beliefs and our behaviour; between our credo and our conduct.

It behoves all of us to take stock and ask ourselves some difficult questions. Do I live a holy life? Am I different from non-Christians in any way? Am I disciplined in keeping God's laws? Am I distinguished by the mark of Christ on my life? Am I dedicated to worshipping him alone?

To those who are truly reborn in Christ, and who put their hand to the plough faithfully, growing in his grace, God has promised rich rewards:

*In all these things we are more than conquerors through
him who loved us.*

Romans 8:37

*Thanks be to God who in Christ always leads us in
triumphal procession.*

2 Corinthians 2:14

*If the Spirit of him who raised Jesus from the dead dwells
in you, he who raised Christ from the dead will give life to
your mortal bodies also through the Spirit that dwells in
you.*

Romans 8:11

It is only the Christians who are prepared to give themselves
to prayer and study, learning to live like Christ and opening
their hearts to the power of the Holy Spirit, who can ever
hope to be effective witnesses to the gospel. And thus they
can be effective healers, by opening the way for the sick and
troubled to find their peace in Christ. As Christians we need
to ask ourselves whether our whole Christian life does
indeed reveal Christ – in our families, at work and among
our friends, neighbours and acquaintances.

A world of need

There is no doubt that there is a need for such a witness, in
our modern, hectic, materialistic world. Nations are caught
up in acrimonious disputes and feuds, made more
threatening because of the weapons and powers available to
them for warfare and terrorism. Individuals are in despair,
lost in their neuroses, depressions and sin. We know how
great is the need for Christ's peace and healing at every
level.

Those suffering individuals are not just "out there" in the world; they are among us, in our churches. We have said over and over again in this book that Christians are not immune from suffering ill health, either physical, mental or spiritual. There is work for Christian healers to do, even when the doctors and psychiatrists have done their best, because the Christian alone can provide the spiritual support which is the final piece of the puzzle, the love that fills the "God-shaped space" in the spirit.

Called to serve

One of God's greatest promises is offered to us when we truly seek his way of holiness: "If my people who are called by my name humble themselves, pray, seek my face, and turn from their wicked ways, then I will hear from heaven, and will forgive their sin and heal their land" (2 Chronicles 7:14). God is calling us to be the mediators of his grace, and he calls us to a life that is different, dedicated, and holy. There are four things that distinguish such lives:

• personal and cooperative prayer

• regular worship – seeking God's presence in our homes, chapels, churches and gatherings

• exercising our God-given gifts, especially witnessing to the power of the gospel

• personal commitment to the fellowship of God's ministering people.

These are choices which are open to all believers. I do not say, "to ordinary Christians", because there are no ordinary Christians. We who live in Christ are extraordinary – we may not be on the Queen's Honours List here on earth, but we are all on the honours list of the King of Kings and Lord of Lords. We have the power to be made whole, to be made holy and to be healed, if we hunger and thirst after righteousness.

It is only in this way that we can become effective witnesses and effective healers: by having a personal relationship with the living Christ; by having a personal experience of the regenerative and sanctifying work of God's love; and by experiencing the power of the Holy Spirit in our lives. Alone we cannot bring one sinner to repentance; we cannot offer forgiveness; we cannot open the eyes of the spiritually blind and we cannot give the gift of faith. We can only point the way to the one who can do all these things. We are called to serve him.

Christian counselling

As a professional psychiatrist, I know the power – and the limitations – of secular counselling. Psychotherapy can and does work wonders for many mental disorders, but as a Christian I know that it cannot reach the deepest needs of the human heart. Only God can do that.

Jesus the counsellor

Jesus suffered all the ills the world could throw at him, and consequently he was the best and most empathetic of counsellors. He shared the burdens of every heart and felt them acutely, yet he remained serene and sympathetic, even when crowds of people made endless demands on his time and energy.

He met individuals face to face and understood the secrets of their hearts – like the Samaritan woman who came to draw water from the well and ended up discussing the deepest issues of her life, or Nicodemus who came to him at night, afraid to be seen. Jesus cured people who came to him for physical healing, but he often touched on their spiritual needs as well; he knew when there was sin to be repented. He counselled the crooked civil servant, the social snob and the rich young man; he even counselled the thief who was dying beside him on the cross. He cured the depression of the two disciples on the road to Emmaus. Whether it was the needs of the handful of men he had gathered to be his friends, or the hunger of the 5,000 who followed him into the countryside, Jesus was always counselling and helping others. For the three years of his public ministry he guided, counselled, taught and encouraged the people around him.

When the disciples were fearful of life without him, Jesus promised that he would send "another counsellor" to teach and guide them as he had done. The word used in John 14:16 is *parakletos*, which literally means "standing beside" – the best possible definition of a counsellor. The one who stands beside us to comfort and counsel us is the Holy Spirit.

The Christian healer

Not every Christian who suffers from mental illness can hope to see a Christian psychiatrist. Does this mean that Christians are unable to receive the holistic cure for which they long? Certainly not, for this is where the pastor and the church fellowship can fill the gap. Working with sensitivity and intelligence, using lessons drawn from psychiatric practice, but under the guidance of the Holy Spirit, Christians can supply the final element of spiritual health. This is not instead of proper medical and psychiatric care, but as well as.

True healing comes from wholeness, and as Christians we can share in the great work of restoring the broken-hearted, the despairing, the lost and the lonely, by bringing them into the light of Christ, the love of God, and the fellowship of the Holy Spirit.

Notes

1 *Jesus Take Me As I Am* by Dave Bryant. Copyright (c) 1978 Thankyou Music

Useful Addresses

ACMHA African Caribbean Mental Health Association
Suite 37
49 Effra Road
Brixton
London SW2 1BZ
020 7737 3603

Acorn Christian Healing Trust
Whitehill Chase
High Street
Bordon
Hampshire GU35 0AD
01420 478121
www.acornchristian.org

Action Mental Health
Mourne House
Knockbracken Healthcare Park
Saintfield Road
Belfast BT8 8BH
02890 403726
www.actionmentalhealth.org.uk

Alcoholics Anonymous
PO Box 1, Stonebow House
Stonebow
York YO1 7NU
01904 644026
www.alcoholics-anonymous.org.uk

Alzheimer's Society
Gordon House
10 Greencoat Place
London SW1P 1PH
020 7306 0606
www.alzheimers.org.uk

ANXIA (The Anxiety Disorders Association)
4 Cheltenham Road
Chorlton-cum-Hardy
Manchester M21 9QN
0161 227 9898

Association for Pastoral Care in Mental Health
St Marylebone Parish Church
Marylebone Road
London NW1 3LT
01483 538936
www.pastoral.org.uk

Association for Post Natal Illness
145 Dawes Road
Fulham
London SW6 7EB
020 7386 0868
www.apni.org

Association of Christian Counsellors
29 Momus Boulevard
Coventry CV2 5NA
0845 124 9569
www.acc-uk.org

British Association for Counselling and Psychotherapy
BACP House
35-37 Albert Street
Rugby CV21 2SG
0870 443 5252
www.bacp.co.uk

British Psychological Society
St Andrew's House
48 Princess Road East
Leicester
LE1 7DR
0116 254 9568
www.bps.org.uk

Carers National Association
20-25 Glasshouse Yard
London EC1A 4JT
0808 808 7777 (Carers' line)
020 7490 8818
www.carersuk.org

Centre for Stress Management
Broadway House
3 High Street
Bromley BR1 1LF
020 8228 1185
www.managingstress.com

Childline
Freepost 1111
London N1 0BR
0800 11 11 (urgent calls)
020 7650 3370
www.childline.org.uk

Chinese Mental Health Association
2nd Floor, Zenith House
155 Curtain Road
London EC2A 3QY
020 7613 1008
www.cmha.org.uk

Churches' Council for Health and Healing
St Luke's Hospital for Clergy
14 Fitzroy Square
London W1P 6AM
020 7388 4954

Compass (Counselling on Merseyside Pastoral & Supporting Service)
25 Hope Street
Liverpool L1 9BQ
0151 708 6688
www.compass-counselling.org.uk

Compassionate Friends (Support for bereaved parents)
53 North Street
Bristol BS3 1EN
0117 966 5202
0845 123 2304 (Helpline)
www.tcf.org.uk

Council for Involuntary Tranquillizer Addiction
Cavendish House
Brighton Road
Waterloo
Liverpool L22 5NG
0151 474 9626

Cruse Bereavement Care
126 Sheen Road
Richmond
Surrey TW9 1UR
020 8939 9530
www.crusebereavementcare.org.uk

Depression Alliance
212 Spitfire Studios
63–71 Collier Street
London N1 9BE
0845 123 2320
www.depressionalliance.org

Eating Disorders Association
First Floor, Wensum House
103 Prince of Wales Road
Norwich NR1 1DW
01603 619090
www.edauk.com

Epilepsy Action (British Epilepsy Association)
New Anstey House
Gateway Drive
Yeadon
Leeds LS19 7XY
0113 210 8800
www.epilepsy.org.uk

Ex-Services Mental Welfare Society (Combat Stress)
Tyrwhitt House
Oaklawn Road
Leatherhead
Surrey KT22 0BX
01372 814600
www.combatstress.org.uk

Fellowship of Hope (Prayer and support network)
42 Foxley Lane
Purley
Surrey CR22 3EE

First Steps to Freedom
1 Taylor Close
Kenilworth
Warwickshire CV8 2LW
01926 864473
0845 120 2916 (Helpline)
www.first-steps.org

For dementia (Dementia Relief Trust)
6 Camden High Street
London NW1 0JH
020 7874 7210
www.fordementia.org.uk

Headway (The Brain Injury Association)
4 King Edward Court
King Edward Street
Nottingham NG1 1EW
0115 924 0800
www.headway.org.uk

Help the Aged
207–221 Pentonville Road
London N1 9UZ
020 7278 1114
www.helptheaged.org.uk

Jewish Association for the Mentally Ill
16a North End Road
London NW11 7PH
020 8458 2223
www.jamiuk.org

Manic Depression Fellowship
Castle Works
21 St George's Road
London SE1 6ES
020 7793 2600
www.mdf.org.uk

Mental Health Foundation
9th Floor, Sea Containers House
20 Upper Ground
London SE1 9QB
020 7803 1100
www.mentalhealth.org.uk

MIND (The Mental Health Charity)
15–19 Broadway
London E15 4BQ
020 8519 2122
www.mind.org.uk

MIND Cymru
3rd Floor, Quebec House
Cowbridge Road East
Castlebridge
Cardiff CF11 9AB
0292 039 5123

National Alliance of Relatives of the Mentally Ill (NARMI)
Tydehams Oaks
Tydehams
Newbury
Berkshire RG14 6JT
01635 551923

National Drugs Helpline (24 hours)
0800 77 66 00

National Phobics Society
Zion Community Resource Centre
339 Stretford Road
Hulme
Manchester M15 4ZY
0870 122 2325
www.phobics-society.org.uk

No Panic
93 Brands Farm Way
Telford
Shropshire TF3 2JQ
01952 590005
www.nopanic.org.uk

Northern Ireland Agoraphobia and Anxiety Society
29–31 Lisburn Road
Belfast BT9 7AA
01232 235170
www.praxiscaregroup.org.uk

OCD Action
Suite 107
22–24 Highbury Grove
London N5 2EA
0870 360 6232
www.ocdaction.org.uk

Parkinson's Disease Society of the UK
215 Vauxhall Bridge Road
London SW1V 1EJ
020 7931 8080
www.parkinsons.org.uk

Relate (Relationship counselling)
Herbert Gray College
Little Church Street
Rugby CV21 3AP
01788 573241
www.relate.org.uk

Rethink (National Schizophrenia Fellowship)
30 Tabernacle Street
London EC2A 4DD
020 7330 9100
www.rethink.org

Richmond Fellowship
80 Holloway Road
London N7 8JG
020 7697 3300
www.richmondfellowship.org.uk

Royal College of Psychiatrists
17 Belgrave Square
London SW1X 8PG
020 7235 2351
www.rcpsych.ac.uk

Sainsbury Centre for Mental Health
134–138 Borough High Street
London SE1 1LB
020 7827 8300
www.scmh.org.uk

Samaritans
The Upper Mill, Kingston Road
Ewell
Surrey KT17 2AF
020 8394 8300
www.samaritans.org.uk

SANE
1st Floor, Cityside House
40 Adler Street
London E1 1EE
020 7375 1002
www.sane.org.uk

SANELINE
2nd Floor, 199–205 Old Marylebone Road
London N1 5QP
0845 767 8000

Scottish Association for Mental Health
Cumbrae House
15 Carlton Court
Glasgow G5 9JP
0141 568 7000
www.samh.org.uk

Seasonal Affective Disorder Association (SADA)
PO Box 989
Steyning BN44 3HG
01903 814942
www.sada.org.uk

Shaw Trust (Helping people back into employment)
Fox Talbot House
Greenways Business Park
Malmesbury Road
Chippenham SN15 1BN
01225 716300
www.shaw-trust.org.uk

Stillbirth and Neonatal Death Society (SANDS)
28 Portland Place
London W1B 1LY
020 7436 7940
www.uk-sands.org.uk

Together (Supporting people with mental health needs)
1st Floor, Lincoln House
296–302 High Holborn
London WC1V 7JH
020 7061 3400
www.together-uk.org

Triumph over Phobia
PO Box 3760
Bath BA2 3WY
0845 600 9601
www.triumphoverphobia.com

True Freedom Trust (Counselling for those struggling with homosexuality and related problems)
PO Box 13
Prenton
Wirral CH43 6YB
0151 653 0773
www.truefreedomtrust.co.uk

Turning Point (For drink, drug and mental health problems)
Unit 3.05, New Loom House
101 Backchurch Lane
London E1 1LU
020 7702 2300
www.turning-point.co.uk

Young Minds
48–50 St John Street
London EC1M 4DG
020 7336 8445
www.youngminds.org.uk

Young Minds Parent Information Service
48–50 St John Street
London EC1M 4DG
0800 018 2138